Promoting
Advanced Access
in
Primary Care

The bucket on the front cover represents the daily load of work we all face. We all have choices as to what our buckets contain. What we do is what we choose to do.

Promoting
Advanced Access
in
Primary Care

A Handbook

for those working in Primary Care
and those who enable and manage them

Thomas S. Warrender

Aeneas

First published in 2002
by Aeneas Press

PO Box 200
Chichester
West Sussex
PO18 OJW
United Kingdom

© 2002, Thomas S. Warrender

Typeset in AGaramond
by Marie Doherty

Printed and bound by
MPG Books
Bodmin
Cornwall
United Kingdom

ISBN: 1-902115-25-2

British Library Cataloguing in Publication Data
A catalogue record of this book is available from the British Library

Warrender, Thomas S.

About the author

Dr Stuart Warrender is a General Practitioner who has worked in March, Cambridgeshire for the last 26 years. He has been substantially involved in the use and education of Advanced Access.

Acknowledgements

This book is dedicated to the staff that has enabled Advanced Access to become a reality at Mercheford House. The exercise of writing this book has confirmed the truth of what I have believed and have been saying for some time: Advanced Access is based on the individual contributions of all practice staff not simply the doctors, and has as much to do with people than processes.

Advanced Access would not have been delivered in Mercheford House without Julie, Eileen, Pauline, Tracy, Sue, Julie, Diane, Barbara, Claire, Leia, Sophie, Tina, Denise, Erica, Helen, Sharon, Patricia, Lynn, Avril, Eamonn, David and John.

Considerable thanks to Dr John Oldham and the National Primary Care Development Team who developed these concepts in the UK and have been responsible for introducing the concept of Advanced Access to thousands of practices.

Thanks also to Dr Leslie Cook and Marjorie M. Godfrey of Dartmouth Hitchcock MC, Nashua, New Hampshire, USA and to Dr Mark Murray of Murray, Tauntau & Associates, Sacramento, CA for developing these thoughts and sharing his wisdom.

Thanks to Agnes for knowing what I wanted to say, and to Anand Kumar for his encouragement and trust.

The publishers are grateful to both Dr Mark Murray and Dr John Oldham for their encouragement and support in making this publication happen.

Contents

Foreword

Advanced Access is a means of improving patient access and choice and, importantly, providing primary care clinicians and managers with greater control over how they manage their own time and deploy resources within their own practices.

When I first introduced the term Advanced Access just over two years ago it was perceived by many as an alien concept in the UK. While many of the ideas supporting Advanced Access were based on ground-breaking work in the USA by Dr Mark Murray, the unifying concept and its application within English general practice was developed my myself and the National Primary Care Development Team during the course of 2000.

The Advanced Access model was promoted as one of the three core programme elements of the Primary Care Collaborative in June 2000, and I well remember the early events when a tin hat and flack jacket would have been more appropriate dress. Changing the atmosphere needed the development of Advanced Access in pioneering practices throughout England. One of the early pioneers was Stuart Warrender and Mercheford House, a practice on the Collaborative.

Stuart and his team not only embraced the ideas for their own patients but became one of the leading lights we invited to demonstrate to others that improved access and improved quality are not only achievable, but intertwined.

During this journey, Stuart has developed a tremendous depth of knowledge about the subject and about the change methodology of PDSAs promoted through the Collaborative. This is amply demonstrated in this book, as is his skill as an excellent communicator. This a good story about real life general practice, and an excellent practical text about Advanced Access.

Dr John Oldham
General Practitioner and Head, National Primary Care Development Team

Preface

You either love it or hate it!

Advanced Access is seen by many as the smart way of achieving patient access target – and by many more as a complete irrelevance. There are doctors and nurses who have made it possible for patients to be seen on the day of their choice – and there are those who claim that this is ill-conceived in principle, impractical in execution and impossible without extra resources.

Othes will admit to the benefits of initial change but are adamant that these changes are not sustainable in the long run. Here is the story of how a group of individuals worked together to enable their patients to see their own doctor on the day of their choice.

This book is structured as follows:

The first two chapters deal with a personal description of how Advanced Access operates in an individual Practice in Cambridgeshire. It is firmly embedded in the culture, resources and issues faced by the patients and staff of one particular Practice.

The aim is to show how it worked in Mercheford House, not to infer that slavishly following the same processes in any other Practice would result in the same success. It simply describes the situation as it exists in the author's Practice.

The four other chapters of the book seek to bring together the wisdom of others so that practice teams may work out for themselves how the same standards of access can be delivered in their particular circumstances.

Advanced Access in Primary Care has been written to encourage, to demonstrate possibilities and to enable the professionals at the coal face of Primary Care to take the initiative to change the quality of their working lives and the services they can provide for their patients.

Who should read this book?

This book has been written to encourage **General Practitioners** and their staffs to regain the enjoyment of their work. Many of us feel out of control. The volume of work flooding into our surgeries overwhelms us and we seem powerless to make a difference.

This is not wholly true; we have choices; we are able to create the space that will improve the quality of care we provide for our patients as and well as the quality of own lives; we can regain the drive, excitement and simple joy that we had when we set out in General Practice many years ago.

All **Practice Staff** should read this book, as one of its main theses is that doctors cannot create the radical change needed without the active support and involvement of the nursing, managerial and administrative staff that work with them. What is required is a complete re-think of the way we *all* work, placing the patient at the centre of what we do and producing safe systems to ensure we deliver what we should in the most efficient and effective manner.

Managers of Primary Care Organisations and Strategic Health Authorities should also read this book, along with political leaders in Health. It has not always been felt that the essence of Primary Care has been understood by these organisations. This book will give some insight into many of the issues faced by General Practitioners and their staff in the delivery of externally generated performance targets.

Patients, too, will find the contents of this book interesting, for it may go some way to explain that many of the failings they may have previously attributed to individual carers are in fact a product of '*the system*', and as such require system solutions.

The aim of this book is to encourage potential solutions, remove the endemic delay for care in General Practice and to increase professional satisfaction at all levels of practice.

Chapter 1

Introduction

Advanced Access can be and has been described in different ways and it is difficult to find an exact definition with which everyone agrees. Delivering Advanced Access in Primary Care, however, certainly involves the following ideas:

- Patients being seen on the day they would like to be seen by the doctor or nurse they would like to see
- *'Doing today's work today'* or, perhaps more importantly, *'Having completed yesterday's work yesterday'*
- The removal of the **delay** is associated with decreased patient and staff satisfaction and a poorer quality of care.

While Advanced Access is delivered through Open Appointment Scheduling, there are other common characteristics of practices that achieve this degree of patient access. The adjacent diagram shows the inter-related characteristics of successful Practices.

The Advanced Access jigsaw

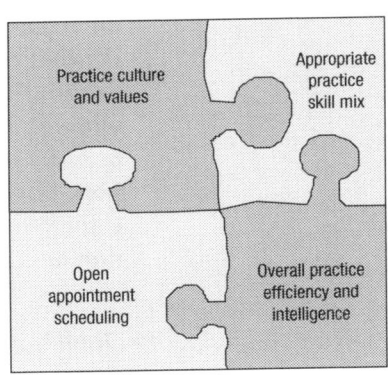

Practice culture and values

Advanced Access cannot be introduced and sustained simply by doctors alone; every member of the Practice needs to be involved. Everyone must understand that this level of access springs, not from the numbers associated with Performance Management, but from the values adopted by the Practice as a whole.

Appropriate Practice skill-mix

Practices require a definite range of staff to meet the access targets we describe. Not every patient requires to see a doctor or nurse; a range of staff members are required to deliver the necessary care. Each team member must work to the limits of his or her skill, knowledge and professional qualification; each must ensure that he or she is doing that which only they, as individuals, are required to do, delegating all else to others. The roll-on from this is that each must know and respect the work of others so that the passage of care between professionals may be safe, seamless and efficient. Every member of staff working in a General Practice is involved in care; each should be developed to make their part more valuable and valued.

Overall Practice efficiency and intelligence

This third pre-requisite for Advanced Access relates to the necessity to know and understand what goes on in the Practice. The use of the word 'intelligence' in this context relates not so much to the IQ of doctors and their staff, but the detailed knowledge of exactly what happens in the organisation as a whole, when it is likely to happen, and work habits and content of all staff. We must understand our patient demand, how it varies in composition between different days of the week and times of the day. We must employ efficient systems that save minutes here and seconds there in order to turn them into precious clinical time. We must reduce handoffs and delays; we should have systems that build on each other in order to reduce the wasted workload associated with duplication. Having patients ring back for information that has not been gathered or shared, or having them return to pick up a prescription or certificate steals clinical time and is totally unproductive.

Open appointment scheduling

This is the vehicle through which Advanced Access is delivered; it is only by having worked off the system backlog, by having done yesterday's work yesterday, that patients can be asked, 'When would you like to see doctor?' Protecting tomorrow's free appointment space by completing today's work today is a fundamental characteristic of Open Scheduling.

It is equally imperative, however, to understand that the ways in which we deal with our backlogs must be intrinsically different to the ways in which we deliver our daily workload.

Why we adopted Advanced Access

As a practice, we did not undertake to deliver Advanced Access to meet externally imposed performance targets, however noble these might have been. We did not undertake this improvement in our quality of care to satisfy the managerial or political yearnings of others, whether at local or national level. Nor did we implement the necessary changes because we felt we 'had to'!

From the other point of view, however, we did not deliver Advanced Access because we knew (or even guessed) how good it would make us feel! Initially, we had no idea of the satisfaction associated with having done today's work today. This was an unexpected, but most satisfying outcome.

The reasons that led us to our action were really embedded in our Practice Values, as identified by our Practice Staff when they completed the Workbook used to develop our Practice Plan for 2001–2003. This leaflet not only produced the content of our Plan in terms of the things we had to do, but also the characteristics, culture and values that would enable our staff to be proud to work at Mercheford House.

In order to be consistent with these values, the doctors had to look at the way they were delivering care and using their staff. The natural outcome was Advanced Access!

> **We did it to be consistent with our values at Mercheford House**
>
> - Patients
>   - We will provide the highest possible quality care to our registered patients
> - Staff
>   - We will respect our staff and develop them to their fullest potential
> - Efficiency
>   - We will be maximally efficient in the way we use our resources.

Current Practice profile

Our Practice shows little difference to the average General Practice throughout UK (or other countries that respect a Primary/Secondary Care Divide). We have perhaps a few advantages around the fact that the practice has had a history of stability of GP partnership. The fact that the doctors have their individual list of patients who consult only their registered doctor at all times – other than when the doctor is on annual leave, is sick or unavailable by arrangement and agreement with his partners. This means that we deliver a continuity of care, and patients always have access to their *own* GP.

Although our premises are a little cramped for everything we would like to do, we do own them and enjoy the freedom that that allows.

The Practice has been engaged at the forefront of many of the activities effecting General Practice in the UK over the last 10 to 15 years, in that we had experience of GP Fundholding, managed Cambridgeshire's only Total Purchasing Pilot and were heavily involved in the formation of our local Primary Care Trust. This has provided an invaluable insight into management and the value of good and bad systems.

> **Practice profile**
>
> - Three partners (in partnership for 26, 16 and 1 years respectively)
> - Individual list system, averaging 2,100 to 2,150 patients each
> - Own our premises
> - 3rd Wave Fundholding Practice
> - Part of a Total Purchasing Pilot
> - Clinical leadership in the PCT
> - Belief that staff are a valuable resource

Practice staff

- Practice manager and part-time assistant
- 3 personal secretaries (30 hrs/wk)
- Repeat prescription clerk
- 1 full-time +3 part-time receptionists
- Fully integrated nursing complement with care assistant
  - Nurses: 37 + 20 (+ 2 x ~4 hrs/wk and as required for annual leave, etc.)
  - Care assistant: 32 hrs/wk
- Two cleaners

A Practice characteristic without which it is very difficult to deliver Advanced Access is a respect for staff. We have sought to demonstrate this in various ways, not least by seriously involving them in the way services are delivered.

In addition to our Practice Attached Community Nursing Staff and Health Visitor, the Practice directly employs the staff shown opposite. How many of them are occupied will be described later, but it is not felt that we are totally distinct to other Practices, though it must be admitted that we did employ new staff and increase the hours of others using GP Fundholding drug savings and contract shifts from Secondary Care Contracts during the Total Purchasing Pilot.

The personal challenge of Advanced Access

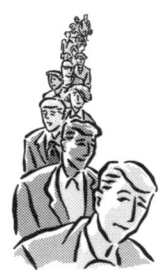

If you go on doing what you are doing now, you are very likely to go on getting the same results as you are getting now!

Having described some of the background to our Practice, and before going on to describe some of the mechanisms we used to deliver Advanced Access in Mercheford House, I should like you to face the Challenge of Change. Put simply, if you are happy doing what you are doing and with the results you are getting, then read no further!

If you are content to have your patients wait 1, 3 or 21 days to see you, then forget it. You will find much with which to disagree – which will give you the perfect excuse to put this book down, never to be read again.

If, however, you are dissatisfied with the outcomes of your Practice Systems and the fixed delays they produce, then perhaps you will learn of ways to change – but beware....

Much of what I write is rubbish! I would reckon that at least half of what you read will be of absolutely no value to you or your Practice. But look out; the other half will be pure gold – exactly the answer you have been seeking. The trouble is, **I do not know the difference!** Only you can work that out – and to do so, you will probably have to read the book in its entirety. Seriously, try to look behind the example, the story or the quip for a truth that you can apply to your own situation, in your unique array of practice circumstances.

Do not look for some form of *Holy Grail*, for there will be nothing here that is not being done much better in some other Practice in UK. It was, however, the systematic adoption and implementation of these ideas that has allowed my partners and me to *do today's work today.*

> When I was speaking with my Practice Manager about Advanced Access and how to explain it to others, she turned to me and said, "It's easy if there are women in your audience."
>
> I looked at her, not knowing of a gender difference in understanding this concept. "What do you mean?"
>
> "It's easy. Tell them about the ironing in the laundry basket, and the shirt or blouse they don't like ironing!" I looked at her for a moment trying to think like a housewife. She came to my aid and dispelled my ignorance. "If you keep up with the ironing after each wash, it's not too bad. If you put off ironing the blouse you don't like doing, then it becomes a chore in that it meets you next time. If you come home to two weeks ironing after a holiday, it's even worse. The secret," she informed me, "is to keep up with the work, and clear the ironing basket on a regular basis – including the shirt you don't like doing! Sometimes," she smiled, "it gets so dry, you have to wash it again!"
>
> Even to my innocent male mind, there seemed a moral here somewhere that was applicable to Advanced Access as well as ironing.

Chapter 2

Access

Advanced Access – Mercheford House style

For the sake of illustration, let us consider the **Patient Parcel Journey at Mercheford House**. Using this analogy, patients present at reception before passing through to professionals who deliver care in one form or another. Patients then leave the building, often after they have made contact with our receptionists again.

One of the things that can go wrong with this journey is that the demand at reception becomes heavier than one would like. Too many parcels are delivered for processing.

Before we start complaining about the apparent ever increasing demand for appointments, let's look at the way many of us train our reception staff. Usually, one of the areas of initial instruction involves teaching our new recruits to say, 'No' to patients requests.

"No, I'm sorry, you can't get an appointment that day."

"No, I'm sorry, all the routine appointments have been used up."

Entry system constraints:

Too many parcels for processing

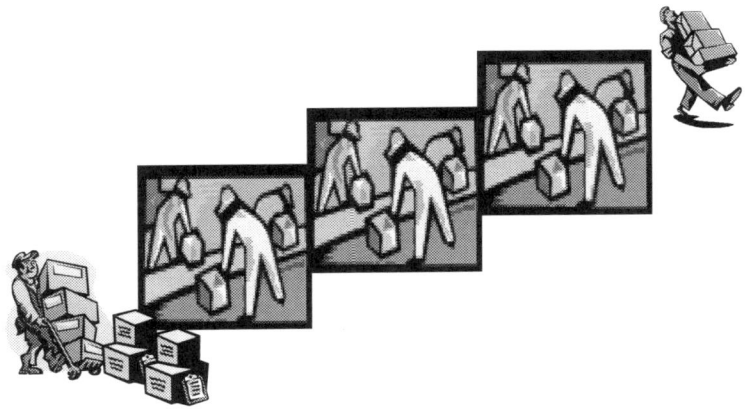

Characteristics of the usual appointment system

- Receptionists are paid to say, 'No' to patients rather than 'Yes'
- Mondays are bad days!
- 'Discussions' anticipated
- Complicated templates based on urgent, routine and special appointment types for each GP
- Necessity to clear yesterday's work first before starting today's
- Fixed delay to see any particular doctor

"No, I'm sorry, Dr Warrender's first free appointment is two weeks on Friday."

"No, I'm sorry….!"

"No!"

Without caricaturing receptionists, it is no surprise that many find it difficult in a job where one uses an apology for one's actions for much of the day.

One thing that we do not have to teach our receptionists is that Mondays are bad days. They learn this for themselves after their first full week of work. Nor do we need to point out to them that if they are going to 'pull a *sickie*', Monday is the day!

Much time is spent teaching new receptionists how to have 'discussion' with patients. Often an experienced receptionist may be seen whispering in the ear of a more junior colleague some advice as to what to say to the patient making a phone request to see their doctor. While this does not always amount to being taught how to lie more pleasantly and effectively, in reality, this is often the case!

The brinkmanship often displayed by receptionists when they 'discuss' the merits of an urgent appointment request with a patient feeling less than wholly well can be something to watch.

"I've told you, all his routine appointments are taken up! Is it urgent that you **must** be seen today?"

"Well, doctor said I should come back if I was not better"

"All I have are urgent appointments. You would need to come and sit till you were seen. Is it **really** that urgent for today?"

This barter often goes on till one of the contestants blinks: the patient, perhaps, lies and shouts, "Yes, it's urgent. I need to be seen today!"

Or the receptionist is very measured in an almost threatening voice, says something like, "OK. I've given you an urgent appointment. You'll just need to wait and take you turn!" She then slams the phone down in the knowledge that she has been beaten by that manipulating patient again!

If, however, she had 'won', she might well have worried the entire week until the patient is seen, just in case she had refused an appointment to someone in need of urgent clinical care.

The reception area can often sound more like a war zone, and gives just about as much job satisfaction.

Another way to make life difficult for our receptionists is to invent a complicated system of red lines, blue line and green line – each having a totally different significance to patients, receptionists, practice managers and GPs!

"But that means that you can only book beneath it if there has been a Monday holiday after the doctor has been on call the night before – except if he is due on annual leave or PCT meeting!" learns a new receptionist from one with longer experience and who has got it wrong more often. Life can become so complicated that receptionists develop their own way through the morass:

"If you call me at 5 minutes before closing time, after the doctor has left, I'll squeeze you in!" Or, "Call me before surgery starts on Wednesday. Ask to speak to me personally."

To say that these activities do not go on would be naive of doctors. The challenge is that the degree to which appointment systems are circumvented or bent depends on their complexity and un-workability. The use of an Advanced Access system, where patients are seen on the day of their choice by the doctor of their choice, can cause many of these issues to disappear.

Receptionists have known for years something that doctors are now only cottoning on to: the problem with most appointment systems is that before a doctor can set about doing today's work he or she must first clear off work that should have been done the day before or the week before! If the patient who has been asked to, "Ring back on tomorrow and I'll fit you in" had only been seen on the day of their first contact, the work would have been done, and a space would have been left in which to do today's work

Another fact known to receptionists is that the delay to see a particular doctor is usually constant. It may be one day to see Dr A for a routine appointment, 3 days for Dr B and 3 weeks for Dr C – but these do not vary a lot. They have been similar as long as Drs A, B and C have worked together. Even with the introduction of Chronic Disease Management Clinics, they have remained the same.

At a system level, this is an important observation, for it means that the Practice is balancing its patient demand with its current resources, only 1, 3 or 21 days too late! Month on month, the doctors are seeing the patients that need to be seen; their workload is in balance – but patients have to wait 1, 3 or 21 days. The system is balanced, but has a fixed delay – but more of this anon.

Patterns of work at reception

One of our early PDSA cycles,[1] concerned the front of house workload. Here we simply measured the number of patients presenting over the course of the day. What is displayed is the mean of two weeks' observations.

The receptionists also counted the number of telephone calls coming in over the course of the day. Both of these activities were then added together to provide some idea of front-of-house activity.

[1] PDSA Cycles. These are simply a form of audit cycles which have special and peculiar qualities. They are described later in Chapter 5. The abbreviation stands for Plan, Do, Study, Act.

Front of house patient workload

Patients calls and presentations compared with receptionist presence

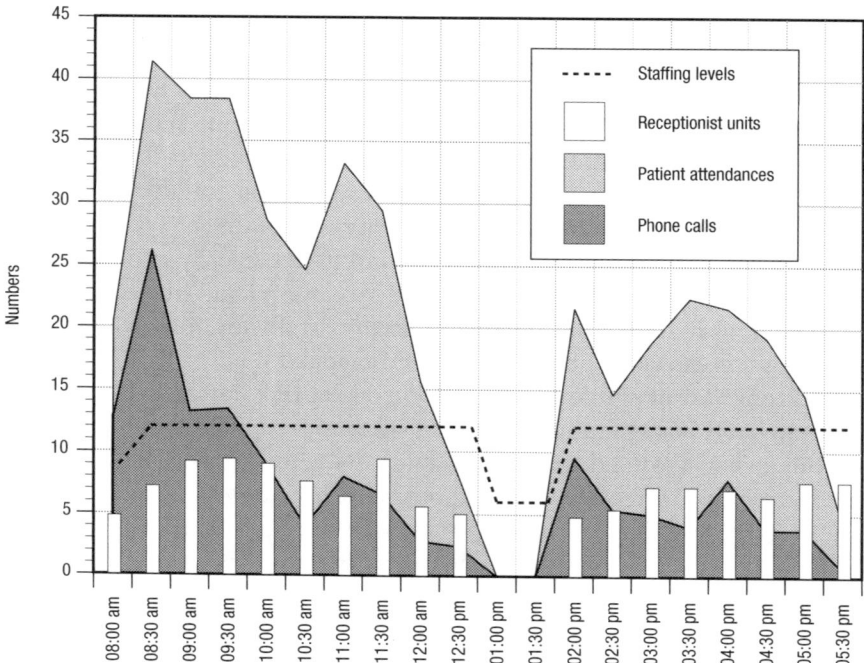

What became obvious was that there were two peaks of work in the morning – one around 8.30 a.m. and another around 11.00 a.m. Both of these were associated with the start of our morning and forenoon surgeries. While the volumes were not as great in the afternoon, a similar bimodal graph was generated.

While this did not amount to a discovery of rocket science proportions, what was fascinating was the fact that the receptionists waited till the second peak at 11.00 a.m. before taking the coffee break! For historical reasons, we waited until it became busy before removing staff from the reception area. This was willingly corrected, to ensure that all reception staff were back at their posts when the demand was highest.

> This principle is by no means limited to receptionists. In one Practice preparing to deliver Advanced Access, it was found that the daily patient demand for appointments fluctuated to such a degree over the days of the week that the number of appointments provided on Monday could not possibly meet Monday's demand. This was not surprising as one of the GPs took his half day on a Monday, the day of highest demand.

By ensuring that there were sufficient doctors present on their busier days, patient demand could be met much more easily and accurately.

We must look again and again at what goes on in our Practices. New doctors joining an existing Practice often inherit the duty patterns of their retiring seniors – as do new secretaries, receptionists and nurses. Their very presence is proof that the practice has changed, and that the old ways are unlikely to suit the current situation. It is one of the basic tenets of Advanced Access that Practice capacity and resources are moved to parallel patient demand where at all possible. Another principle is to move demand from one time and space to another to match capacity wherever this is possible.

Front of house workload

- Make sure all staff are present at the busiest time
- If you cannot move the staff, then move the work to slacker times
- Cross-train staff to ease bottlenecks when they occur
- Consider a 'baskets only till'
  - Checking patients in
  - Issuing repeat prescriptions
- This applies to all staff

Simple appointment theory

While many of us have addressed the intricacies of our appointment system on a regular basis, outcomes have usually involved the moving our existing lines or the creation of new appointment categories. There are, however, three main types of appointment systems:

Basic types of appointment systems[2]

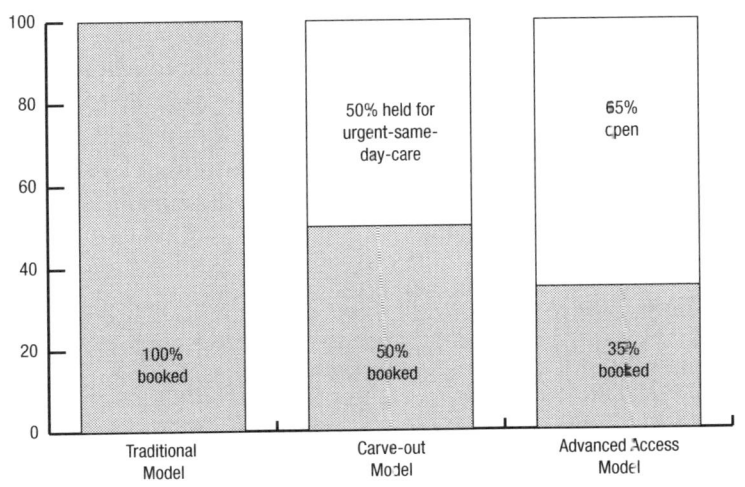

[2] *Same Day Appointments: Exploding the Access Paradigm*, Mark Murray MD, MPA and Catherine Tauntau BSN, MPA, *Family Practice Management*, September 2000, pp. 45–50 (www.aafp.org) http://www.aafp.org/fpm/20000900/45same.html

Traditional Model

The first model is characteristically composed of a simple list of patients and times. As patients present, their names are added to the end of the list. There is no structure, and patients are seen in chronological order.

Systems like this are usually saturated, and the appointment delay in adding patients to the end of the queue may be considerable. If a patient develops a more serious condition, and can convince the receptionist that it is serious, they will classically be 'squeezed in', added as an 'extra' or somehow succeed in super-saturating an already full appointment schedule. This ensures that workflow is seldom regulated, where the finishing time of the professional varies and cannot be predicted from day to day.

Doctors tend not to allow the use of this Traditional Model, but are quite happy for their nursing colleagues to suffer the effects of such a situation.

Carve-out Model

This model can protect both ill patients and the over-worked professionals:

- An estimation is made – either prospectively or retrospectively – of the number of patients who are likely to demand appointments 'on the day'. This may vary according to the day. For example, the *urgent line* may be higher on a Monday than on the other days of the week in order to reflect the varying demand made by patients.
- While this ensures that sufficient space is kept for those who are ill (and can convince the receptionist that they are ill), patients with problems seen to be 'routine' are pushed into the future. The doctor or nurse is happy that he or she has seen everyone who has a problem that must be dealt with today – and who has convinced the Receptionist of this! – but patients (or receptionists) who have made a mistake in the classification of their problem are made to wait the standard delay for a routine appointment.

How often has a doctor seen a patient on Thursday with severe bronchitis? When enquiring, the harassed GP finds that she admits to having developed this over the previous weekend.

Guiltily and defensively, he enquires why she had not sought medical care earlier and he reminds her once more that she has a weak heart.

"Oh, I did, doctor. Honest, I tried to see you. Like you told me last time, I phoned up last Monday morning to see you, but you only had urgent appointments left. Than nice young lady at the front desk told me that I could have an appointment if I was really urgent. I did not want to stop someone with a really serious matter from seeing you.' The patient smiles comfortingly as the doctor sighs, having shrunk in stature somewhat.

It is fascinating; not only has the patient been made to wait for necessary treatment and the doctor been made to be less than proud of the care system over which he presides, but it cost more to treat Mrs. Jones for she ends up using double the strength of antibiotics and perhaps a few more diuretics than he would have prescribed had she been seen on Monday!

In an Advanced Access system, patients are able to see the doctor of their choice on the day of their choice, with the resulting good feelings – and cost savings!

Advanced Access Model

The fundamental characteristic of the Advanced Access Model is that one is up to date with the work! Today's appointment sheet shows free space – for all yesterday's work has been done yesterday. We are free to wait for today's work, knowing that we have the resources to meet it. Receptionists are able to enjoy the incredulity in the voices – and the sound of their jaws hitting the table – of their former opponents when they say, "You mean I can see doctor today?"

There is not a lot more to say about this model. It works! It's great! Everybody wins!

Note that there will always be some degree of backlog. By this we mean that there are always patients whose appointments require being booked in advance. These might include the following:

- Definite follow-up of patients with specific acute problems, e.g. Mrs Jones with her acute bronchitis who we might not have been asked to come back had she been seen at the start of her illness!
- Patients (most of us) who hold diaries and need to plan out lives.
- Work that can be planned and anticipated, such as minor operations and six week postnatal checks.

From a certain perspective, backlog is neither good nor bad, but neutral. It is wholly acceptable as long as it can be managed and does not fill up the daily space necessary to see today's patients today.

Our Practice routinely measures this backlog in terms, not only of the number of pre-booked appointments, but in the number of days necessary to work off the backlog (see later). What is interesting is that this, too, is constant.

Workflow and backlog

It is vital that the difference between normal Practice workflow and backlog be understood and differentiated from each other.

Workflow relates to the rate at which, and the total number of, patients are seen by any one clinician and usually remains fairly constant, unless special circumstances exist. Where this might alter is where partners leave abruptly and the residual work has to be shared between the remaining partners.

Workflow and backlog

- Workflow is usually constant
  - Relates to the number of patients you see in a week/month/year
  - Does not vary much indicating that demand and capacity are really in balance
  - Demand is finite, and can be predicted
  - Backlog and workflow improvement should be approached differently

While the total work a single Practice may face may have altered, the individual workload of the GPs has not. This is evidenced by the annual or monthly consultation figures held by many Practices. They are fairly constant. This in turn indicates that most of us work in stable situations where demand is satisfied by our resources – albeit 1, 3 or 21 days too late! Month on month, there is balance between our demand and supply, allowing for the system delay with which we have chosen to operate.

Further, those Practices who have delivered Advanced Access can support the counter-intuitive notion that in General Practice demand does not increase as we remove the delay.

As breast surgeons who run specialised Breast Units have stated, seeing patients more quickly does not result in an increase in the incidence or prevalence of breast cancer or problems. A similar state of affairs is true in Primary Care.

What is important to understand, however, is that the way we manage our normal work throughout should not be the way to work off our backlog. ***Both must be approached differently.***

Assessment of Practice backlog

When contemplating the possibility of providing an Advanced Access service, it is important to make as realistic an assessment of true backlog as possible.

This is not as difficult as it seems, and includes the following:

- The average number of pre-booked appointments
- The number of patients who misuse the urgent/routine differentiation when they made their appointment
- The number of patients who would like to have seen their own GP on a day different to that on which they did
- It is also important to factor in the work that is subsequent to patients seeing their doctor in this way. Doctors, following initial consultations often refer patients for blood tests, require their secretaries to type letters referring them to specialist colleagues, etc. All these activities constitute backlog.

Medical backlog should be measured in the same units as the delay. One measure of delay might be that defined by Mark Murray[3] and related to the days that might be taken to work off the backlog. The translation between number of booked doctor appointment to days delay is simple:

$$\text{Backlog} = \frac{\text{(Number of pre-booked appointments + consequential appointments)}}{\text{Number of appointments offered per day}}$$

It must be remembered that not all backlog is bad. Some Practices have taken the principle of being seen on the day of request to the extreme in that they do not accept requests for appointment except on the day – or even the morning or afternoon – of the appointment. Appointments can always be had on the day, but the time of day cannot be guaranteed till the day. There may also be little assurance that the appointment will be with the doctor of the patient's choice.

In a world where time planning is important, this cannot be seen as an optimal norm – but may be a successful means to and end.

Resources vs. demand

Traditionally, when changes are required of General Practice, there is an immediate cry for extra resources. While there may occasionally be truth in this claim, it is by no means the necessary

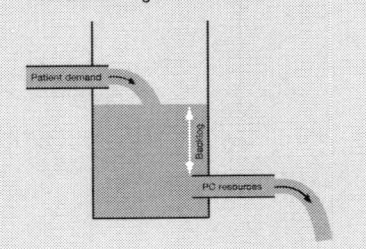

Workflow and backlog

- Backlog not difficult to assess
  - All booked future appointments with the 'knock on' work this creates in the Practice
  - Includes patients who misuse the urgent/routine differentiation
  - Measurable by the number of patients who would have liked to have seen GP sooner
- Can be removed by a **one-off exercise**
- Backlog = $\dfrac{\text{No. pre-booked appointments}}{\text{Average no. of patients seen/day}}$
- Not all backlog is bad

[3] *Same-Day Scheduling,* Helen Lippman, *Hippocrates,* February 2000, pp. 49–53. (www.hippocrates.com) http://www.hippocrates.com/archive/February2000/02features/02openaccess.html

Demand vs. resources

- At an individual level, the volume of Practice work faced by a GP has been, is and will be generally constant
- Demand can be shaped
- Resources are managed well
- Before requesting more resources make what we have maximally efficient

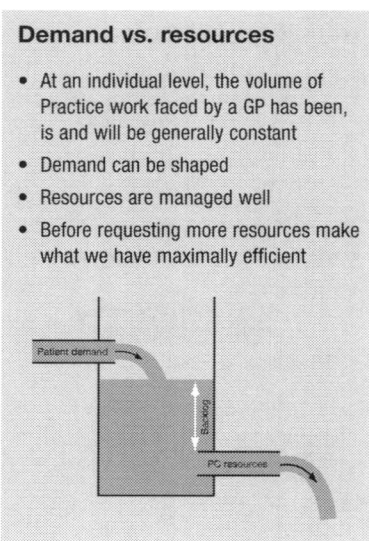

norm. The delivery of an Advanced Access system does not, of itself, require any more resources – though it may need *different* resources. Whether a GP balances his care delivery on a monthly, weekly of daily basis, the resources in terms of people and time are the same. All that is necessary is the clearing of the backlog. Once this has been cleared, all that is required is that he or she works at the same pace as before.

Under Advanced Access, life may become less demanding; for there is evidence that there can be up to a 10–15% reduction in the demand for appointments. In addition, demand can be shaped and resources managed to provide a reduced mismatch of supply to demand. It must certainly be the case, that before blanket requests for more resources for Primary Care are allocated to meet Advanced Access standards, a careful examination of the use of current resources ought be made.

Experience in both Primary and Secondary Care would prove that it is vision and the will to change that have driven change and deliver improvement, rather than the injection of more money. It has been true that money has followed such improvements as it has become possible to deliver even more work, but the original efficiency and re-engineering improvements did **not** require money.

Removing the backlog

Having identified the backlog in our individual Practice Systems, consideration must be given as to how it is going to be worked off.

Method 1: Give it to someone else to do

Remove the backlog – Method 1

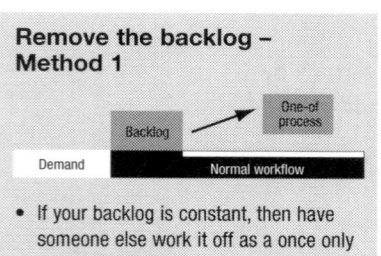

- If your backlog is constant, then have someone else work it off as a once only exercise
- Then meet the reduced demand on a same-day basis

This method uses one-off sums of money to pump prime the system. Having carefully defined the size of the work entailed, application might be made to one's respective Primary Care Organisation with an estimate of the amount of doctor, nurse and secretarial time deemed necessary to work off the backlog identified. The deal would be that having worked it off, having drained the cistern, so to speak, the Practice would agree to see patients on the day of their choice from then onwards.

It should be noted that Practices who pursue and deliver by this means will enjoy the 10–15% reduction in patient demand for appointments, thereby working not only smarter but less hard.

Method 2: Work harder!

Practices on both sides of the Atlantic have gone down this road. They have simply worked off their backlog by working harder. They have provided more appointments, longer hours, more surgery sessions to clear their demand and have reached a point when they have made it a principle of their care that their patients see the doctor of their choice on the day of their choice. They then go on to enjoy the associated reduction in their workload.

Remove the backlog – Method 2

- Increase you personal workload to clear the backlog as a one of process
- Then meet the reduced demand on a same-day basis

Method 3: Work smarter

This third method is the method of choice, for it displays an understanding of the Advanced Access Jigsaw with which this chapter opened.

This scenario involves the systematic and planned shift of work from the GP to other care professionals within the Practice. This principle is called *diverting from the constraint*, though when it was put into practice at Mercheford House, all we thought we were doing was shifting work from the overworked doctor to the nurses! Such was our innocence!

Remove the backlog – Method 3

- Start by deflecting the demand, work at the same pace and clear the backlog at the same time
- Then meet the reduced demand on a same-day basis

What in effect happened was that we gradually informed patients that, as doctors, we did not 'do' high blood pressure any more, and moved our patients to our trained chronic disease nurses. This was in order that we could make time to see patients on the day on which they wanted to be seen. This shift included the routine management of our patients with asthma, diabetes, etc.

It was at this time – before we knew what Advanced Access was – that we began to realise that we had free routine appointments on certain days of the week. While initially we began to wonder if our patients still loved us, trusted us or wanted to see us, the fact of the matter was that on a weekly basis, we were balancing our supply with our patient demand. In fact, the presence of free appointments indicated that we were providing an excessive supply of consultations!

As a consequence, as soon as the backlog had been removed, we went on to enjoy the same reduction in workload as others who had employed other methods – but without the feeling that it had come through money from outside sources or our increased work. We had the satisfaction of having done it 'our way'!

Appointments before and after Advanced Access

The figure below demonstrates what can happen as a Practice moves from a Carve-out to an Open Access appointment.

Classically, we like to think that there are two types of appointments, urgent and routine. After a moment's thought, however, this is a gross simplification.

Within the group normally called urgent, there are two distinct types:

- **True urgent appointments**
  These are patients who develop urgent problems that must be dealt with on the day they develop. They include broken legs, acute infections, painful abdomens, etc. The incidence and prevalence of these conditions are constant, irrespective of the type of appointment system operated.

- **False urgent appointments**
  Patients who fall into this category are those who have what are in reality routine matters, for which they are not prepared

Appointments and Advanced Access

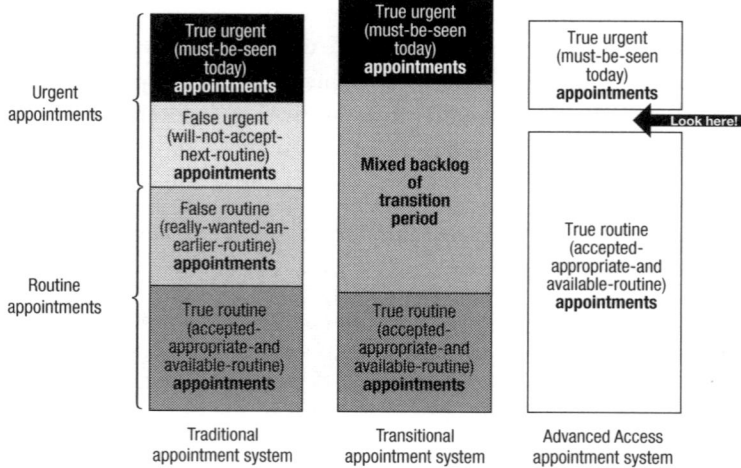

to wait for a normal routine appointment. These are patients who argue or manipulate their way to getting an appointment on the day they wish.

This type of appointment type does relate to the appointment system used, and is greater in the Carve-out Model.

Similarly, when considering routine appointments, the same divisions apply:

- **True routine appointments**
  Patients may be said to have taken a true routine appointment when they are given an appointment on the weekday of their choice, for example, patients who request an appointment for, say, Wednesday, and are given one on Wednesday.

- **False routine appointments**
  On the other hand, patients who request an appointment for Wednesday, but who have to make do with one on Friday fall into the group of false routine appointments. These must be included when assessing Practice backlog.

When the date comes to implement Advanced Access, an interim period is often encountered where a mixed appointment situation is in place. Here, the number of true urgent appointment requests remains constant – Advanced Access has no direct effect on the numbers of broken legs, acute infections, painful abdomens! Equally, there is no increase in the number of patients requesting true routine appointments. Any difference that occurs reflects the number of false routine and false urgent appointments. The number of appointments in this group reflects the Practice backlog; hence the importance of making as accurate an assessment as possible.

After the interim period by which the backlog has been cleared, the Practice will enjoy the 10–15% reduction in workload already described.

The Mercheford House version of Advanced Access appointment scheduling

While there are minor variations between the partners, the general guidelines given to our receptionists include the following:

- Receptionists are no longer required to debate with our patients as to whether an urgent or routine appointment is required. The delay associated with routine appointments has been removed and the distinction between the two appointment types gone for good.

- Patients are currently able to book up to four weeks in the future. Having measured our demand, we feel that it is possible to allow this without encountering the feared blocking of future appointment schedules. Some Practices, especially in the early days of their experience, have reduced this period to one or two weeks. There is no magic length of time. Our belief is that it is as important for patients to be able to plan their lives and use their diaries as it is for members of the medical profession. As we will demonstrate later, we have not been over-run by these arrangements.

- When a doctor is on annual leave, sick or away from the Practice for any other reason, the week of his return is kept totally free of appointments – except for the first four slots, so that he has work to do when he starts his day. Because he has returned to a free appointment schedule, he will be able to see all those patients who wish to see him on the day of their choice. Patients who have requested appointments during his leave are told to phone back during the week he returns when they will be seen on the day of their choice. By this means, no backlog of work is created during his absence or following his immediate return.

  Because of the strength of our individual list system, most patients with routine medical issues will postpone their appointments till their own doctor returns from leave. Patients with problems that cannot wait are seen by the remaining two GPs.

- We encourage our receptionists to use the simplified appointment areas freely. Each of the three doctors prefers slightly different ways of working, and where any excess numbers of patients should be placed, but these are only minor. All three will see patients on the day of their choice, clearing their work on a daily basis.

- As may be seen from the diagram opposite, the 'lines' have disappeared and there is no distinction made in terms of appointment types.

- Our receptionists are encouraged to make sensible decisions and to communicate with the doctors. For example, if their perception of a patient and his or her situation is such that an exception is required to be made, and a patient requires to be 'squeezed in' between existing appointments, or added to the end of a surgery session, she should make this decision on the facts available – but inform the doctor concerned. She is also

Simplified appointment template

	Previous system	Current system	
08:00 am			08:00 am
08:30 am			08:30 am
09:00 am	Routine	Appointments	09:00 am
09:30 am			09:30 am
10:00 am	Urgent		10:00 am
10:30 am			10:30 am
11:00 am			11:00 am
11:30 am	Urgent	Appointments	11:30 am
12:00 pm	Very urgent		12:00 pm
12:30 pm			12:30 pm
01:00 pm			01:00 pm
01:30 pm			01:30 pm
02:00 pm			02:00 pm
02:30 pm			02:30 pm
03:00 pm			03:00 pm
03:30 pm	Urgent		03:30 pm
04:00 pm		Appointments	04:00 pm
04:30 pm	Routine		04:30 pm
05:00 pm			05:00 pm
05:30 pm	Very urgent		05:30 pm
06:00 pm			06:00 pm
06:30 pm			06:30 pm

encouraged to keep her eye on the number of home visits the doctor has at the end of surgery, and to keep him informed as to any developing situation.

- Our receptionists are encouraged to feel empowered by the Advanced Access system of which they are a fundamental part, and to enjoy saying, 'Yes' to patients.

Fears of being over-run by Advanced Access

While it is an obvious and understandable fear that Advanced Access will simply open the floodgates of patients' demand, this

Average weekly appointment pattern (all doctors)

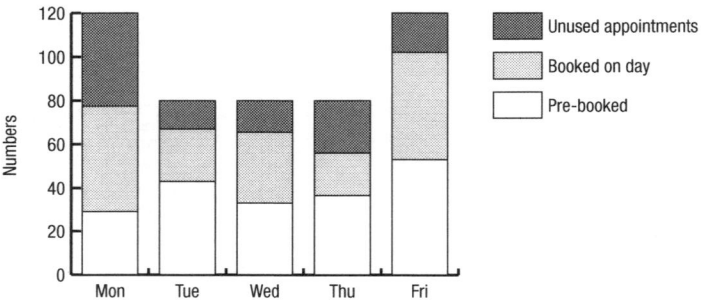

has not proved true over the 18 months I have operated the system. The results of the following two PDSA Cycles would support this.

Over three weeks in the autumn of 2001, we audited the daily appointments for all three doctors in terms of:

1. those that had been made prior to the day in question
2. those that had been made on the day
3. those that had been left unused.

Note these are average figures. Whilst in one week, one of us had extra patients on at least one day, the thrust of the data would indicate that we were supplying our patient demand with the resources at hand.

The other big fear is that our future appointments might be blocked. The diagram opposite demonstrates that this problem did not arise.

On a regular basis, each Saturday morning to be precise, a count is made of all appointments that have been pre-booked for the following four weeks.

Translating the raw count into number of days of work necessary to clear all appointments, a backlog varying between one to just under three days has been found. Future appointments are not flooded by delivering Advanced Access.

What Advanced Access will NOT do!

Open Scheduling and Advance Access is not the answer to all the problems faced in Practice.

- If an appointment system is poorly designed in terms of number or times of appointments offered to patients, these issues required to be addressed before implementing a new system.

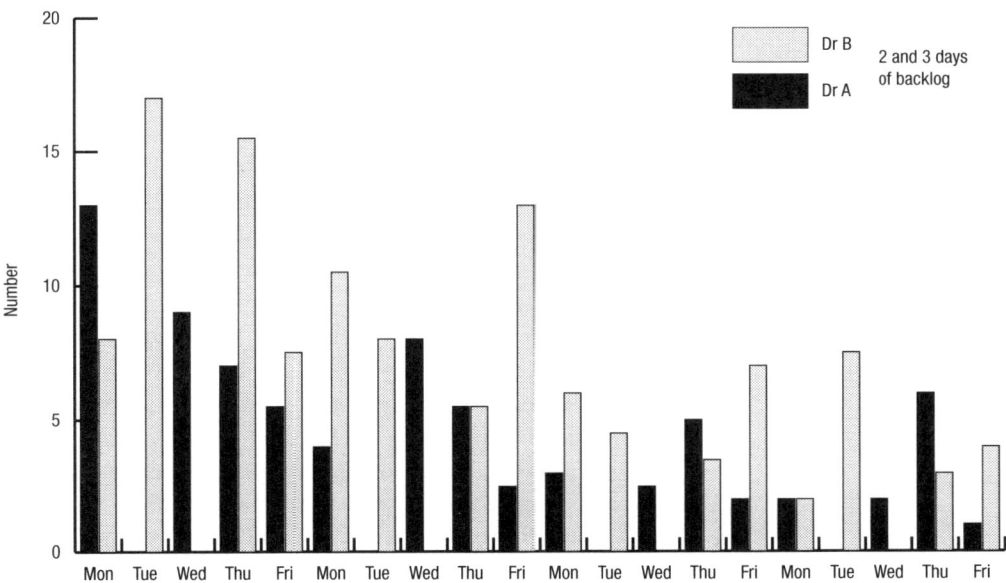

Future pre-booked appointments over the next four weeks

- Poor planning for holidays where several doctors or other key members of staff go off on leave at the same time is not conducive to efficient working of any Practice, and will certainly not be corrected by Advanced Access. Contingency plans need to be made for sudden illness of partners, even if this is only a list of ways and places to locate locums!

- Issues around heart-sink patients will not be tackled by Advanced Access. Personally, I have not found the apparent increase in ease of seeing a doctor make this problem worse – and there are other ways to deal with it and help these unfortunate people.

- The work caused by trivial and inconsistent consultation will not be addressed by Advanced Access principle – solutions for these issues lie with the doctor and his consistent handling of patients who so present. As we have said before, doctors have the patients they deserve!

- Extending this point, in situations of truly unrealistic demand, where Practices are a doctor down, or waiting for a replacement, some other more appropriate solution must be found, either in the form of a new GP or a change in the way the existing doctors work with their nursing staff

> **What Advanced Access will not do!**
>
> - It will not automatically deal with a disorganised Practice:
>   - A poorly designed appointment system
>   - Poor planning for holidays and sickness
>   - Heart-sink patients who take up more than their planned consultation time
>   - Trivial and inconsistent consultations
>   - Unrealistic patient demand
>   - Doctors who are not prepared to delegate to trained colleagues
>   - Doctors who ask patients to make appointments on their busy days

and nurse practitioners. Situations like this are uncommon, for Practices normally seem to work in a situation of constant delays, i.e. it takes 1, 3 or 21 days to see a doctor. Such a Practice is in balance in terms of its capacity and demand and would benefit from the Advanced Access approach.

- Advanced Access is much easier to operate when doctors – and nurses, for that matter – are able to delegate to each other. Some doctors insist on seeing all (or many) of their hypertensives, asthmatics and diabetics, for example. By so doing, they never have enough time to see the patients who require their services quickly – without having to over-saturate their appointment schedules. By delegating work to others in a planned and controlled way, space can be easily found to see those that wish to see the doctor of their choice on the day of their choice.

- This principle also applies to the appropriate work that doctors keep. For example, having space to see patients on the day they wish, is made a lot easier if GPs do not ask their patients to attend for follow-up appointments on days when they know they will be busy, for example Mondays and Fridays. Demand – especially doctor-generated demand – can be managed and transferred to days that are lighter.

The ways in which doctors work

Sometimes, the behaviour of doctors can be a stumbling block to the running of an efficient appointment system. In a recent PDSA study looking at the delay associated with the time a doctor started his surgery and the delay associated when he saw his last patient of that sessions, three sets of characteristics were found:

1. Dr B started on time and finished on time. Not only was he organised enough to get to the surgery on time, the periodicity with which he saw patients seemed to suit his style of working. Patients were seen on time and he was kept busy.
2. Dr A, on the other hand, consistently started late – sometimes for good reasons, but often not. Having started late, he finished late; but here again, although his appointment duration was slightly longer than Dr B's, he tended to finish as late as he started, indicating that his problems lay not in the length of his appointments, but in the fact he did not start his surgeries on time.
3. Dr C, however, was another kettle of fish. Not only did he not start on time, but he consistently saw his 12.00 p.m. patient at

12.45 p.m. This indicated that his appointment durations did not suit his way of consulting. He consistently used more time when seeing patients; his waiting room bay was always well populated compared to those of Drs A and B, something which frequently generated patient comment.

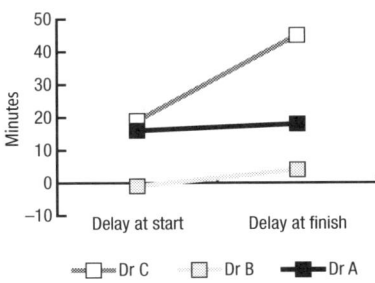

A tale of three doctors

Delay in starting and finishing

The solution for Dr A was to start on time, while for Dr C, this was not sufficient – he needed to lengthen the duration of his appointments to suit his manner of practice. This did not result in his seeing more patients, or working longer hours; it simply meant that the previous patients who had been given a 12.00 p.m. appointment and who waited till 12.45 p.m. before he or she was seen, were now asked to present at 12.45 p.m. and were seen on time.

Advanced Access provides an opportunity to look at all these issues. Appropriate change in the behaviour of GPs added to the increased quiet of the receptions area and providing a waiting area that is less busy and noisy, with perhaps only one patient waiting to see each doctor has a knock-on effect. This is much more conducive to patients coming to the surgery rather than asking for house calls, and generally improves the patient experience.

The calculation

There is a calculation[4] which represents the number of approaches patients in General Practice make to their doctors on a daily basis. This appears to be independent of locality or even country.

It would appear that 0.7 to 0.8% of our patients attempt to contact us on a daily basis.

It then becomes easy to calculate the number of appointments we require to offer patients on a weekly or daily basis.

The weekly number of appointments required to be distributed over the week in such a way as to allow for the daily fluctuation in local demand. This can be calculated using PDSA methodology. The precise number of appointments may be kept constant over the week with the apparent effect of creating 'free space' or may be shaped more closely to the measured demand.

[4] *Same-Day Scheduling*, Helen Lippman, *Hippocrates*, February 2000, pp. 49–53. (www.hippocrates.com) http://www.hippocrates.com/archive/February2000/02features/02openaccess.html

The calculation

- Between 0.7% to 0.8% of your patients contact you each day
- Number of contacts =

$$\frac{\text{list size} \times 0.008 \times 7}{\text{No. of days worked}}$$

- Ensure this number of appointments, distributed over the week in line with local daily Practice fluctuations as calculated using PDSA cycles.
- Appointment templates need to be altered reflecting the increased demand created when doctors (and other clinical staff) are not on leave or sick.

The results of applying the calculation to my own Practice list suggested that I was probably offering more appointments than I needed.

> The findings here indicated that I had free appointments, especially on a Thursday. While many of my colleagues I met at PCT meetings were complaining of over-work, I kept quiet, secretly worrying that my patients did not love me any more, or that they had stopped trusting me with their problems! In effect what had been happening was that I had satisfied their demand for appointments.

A second outcome of performing the calculation was that I could safely standardise all my appointments to 7½ minutes each, or as I prefer to state, 8 patients an hours, thereby allowing for some longer consultations as dictated by patients' problems. This made it easier for our reception staff.

Personal results of the calculation

- Capacity exceeded demand
  - (the reason for my pressure was always putting back yesterday's work)
- Appointment times were standardised to 7.5 minutes
  - (Except when the pressure is on, and when patients are asked to come at a specific time)
- Patients who needed more time were given specific appointments
  - (Often booked as 'Last Patient' at 5.30 p.m.)

Please note that in the Mercheford House version of Advanced Access, every patient is given a specific appointment time. The only exception to this is on the relatively few occasions when the pressure is on. After the 'fire breaks' have been filled, patients are sometimes invited to attend at, say, 5.30 p.m. Only on these occasions will they have to wait to be seen. This is because one of our local pharmacies closes at 6.30 p.m., and we try to give the patient as much time as possible to obtain any necessary prescriptions.

If specific patients are known to require longer appointments, they are not seen in normal surgery time, but special times are given. This also holds true for medical examinations, which are usually performed on Saturday mornings before an urgent surgery by the doctor on duty that morning.

Managing people constraints

Continuing the idea of the parcel journey through Mercheford House – or any other Practice for that matter – we found that after patients passed through the reception process, there were further delays within the systems that impeded their care.

When these were explored, it was apparent that patients were seeing the wrong care professional. The constraint was usually the doctor, on whom much of the work fell.

The figure below was felt to reflect the situation where everything seemed to pass to the GP.

Early bottleneck in the parcel journey

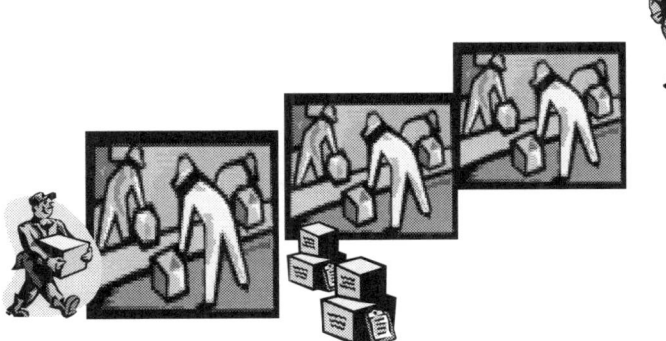
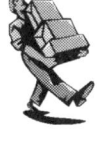

This led to a general examination of the work that staff undertook, and resulted in the concept of the **daily bucket of work**!

All of us, whether manager, receptionists, nurses, secretaries or doctors can cope with a daily amount of work – a bucket of work per day. Many of us, however, have been too busy to see what constitutes our bucket of work or to examine what it contains, and whether it contains work that is appropriate to the individual. Often staff – and doctors – inherit the buckets of their predecessors, and do not have the time or inclination to examine its contents to ensure that they are still what patients need.

When we look into our buckets of daily work, we will usually find that space is being occupied by objects which have gathered through the years and which ought not to be there. We find, for example, the following:

Managing system constraints

Yesterday's work

Perhaps the largest object that takes up space in our buckets is the work we should have done yesterday – or even last week!

When contemplating Advanced Access, the subject of backlog must consume most of one's attention. It must be accurately assessed and addressed in one of the three methods already described.

The daily bucket of work

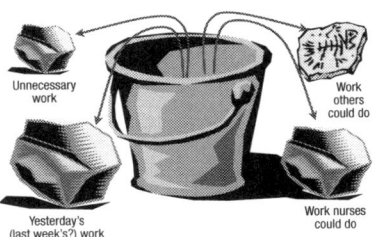

Work that nurses can do

As far as a GP is concerned, the next greatest problem in trying to do the work we do best is to identify the work that should be shifted to our nursing colleagues – not only because it creates clinical space for doctors to see patients on the day they wish to be seen, but because, in many instances, nurses are able to do them better than we can.

Work that others can do

This space, time and resource-occupying stone relates to nurses as well as GPs. All clinical staff must regularly examine their work to ensure that they are only doing that which requires their qualification, training and skills. If the piece of work can be done by someone with lesser qualifications, then it should be handed over in a planned way to the more appropriate person. This, in terms of GPs and nurses, ensures that each only does that for which one requires a medical or nursing degree.

Unnecessary work

The last area that needs scrutiny is the work that all of us regularly undertake that is not required. This extends from clinical staff to everybody working in the Practice. It refers to:

- The duplication of information gathering
- Storing information in places other than the official site, thereby making retrieval difficult if not impossible
- Seeing patients too often for unnecessary follow up.

> I remember working in a Practice where one of the partner's Monday morning surgery was booked months ahead of time with a series of elderly patients with hypertension who presented for their monthly check-up. These appointments were at five-minute intervals from 9.00 a.m. to 10.45 a.m. The doctor concerned had a fairly easy morning to start his week! That would never happen now; or would it? Before we answer, let's look at the things we do to ensure that there is not an equivalent.

Clear the buckets

A good place to start preparing to implement Advanced Access might be to clear all our daily buckets of work that should not have been there in the first place.

We need to find out what actually happens in our Practices

This might be a larger job than we first think. What we think happens is not always the current practice. Ideas that were put in place some time previously often get changed by staff. Sometimes the ideas never did work, and our staff were afraid to tell us for fear of upsetting the doctor whose 'baby' the notion was. Perhaps the idea worked initially, but was changed in the light of experience. We need to find out exactly what goes on using direct questioning, data collection and process mapping techniques.

We need to study what the GPs in the Practice are doing, and whether this is appropriate. Of the many things we do, a number might be less than efficient, and should be given to others.

We need to study what is done by our nurses. The treatment room is often the last common dumping ground that collects all sorts of mixed work, some of which is both appropriate and efficient, but much of which is both inappropriate and inefficient, and can safely be transferred to a less well trained individual.

Since we have introduced our Practice Care Assistant, it has been a pleasure and a humbling experience to see the number of Practice and former nursing tasks that have been delegated to her, after in-house training. Patient and staff acceptance has been high and she has 'grown' with the job.

The last area that needs to be studied in terms of GP and nursing consultations relates to work that does not need to be done, or does not require an appointment to do it.

We need to be constantly reviewing our clinical protocols, altering the follow-up periods in the light of modern evidence-based medicine; what was clinically correct and appropriate even a few years ago needs revision in the light of our greater current knowledge.

Collecting this information is not always as easy as it sounds. One certainly has got to pose the question before the knowledge is gained, and even then it is difficult; questions need to be clear and specific.

Sources of information should include our patients, staff and our spouses, who often seem to see things in our Practice life that we miss!

It is important, as with PDSA Cycle, that when a question is posed, one does something with the answer! The source should also be acknowledged

> **Let's clear the bucket!**
>
> - Find out what actually happens in your Practice
> - Study work patterns and flows
>   - What actually happens in your Practice?
>   - Things that only doctors can do
>   - Things that only nurses can do
>   - Things that others can do
>   - Things that do not need to be done at all!

> **What actually happens in your Practice?**
>
> - It is impossible to know unless you ask – and even then it is difficult!
> - Questions need to be clear and specific – normally only one can be answered at a time
> - Ask your patients, staff, partners and spouse
> - ALWAYS do SOMETHING with the results!

and the appropriate member of staff attributed with any good idea that is forthcoming.

What do nurses do as well as (meaning better than!) doctors?

> **Work that nurses can do as well as doctors (better than?)**
>
> - Conditions that are managed by protocols and require regular follow-up
> - Chronic disease management
>   - Asthma, COPD, diabetes, hypertension, IHD, leg ulcers, pill, skin conditions, etc.
> - Minor Ailments Clinics

Nurse training is fundamentally different to that of doctors, and they have a great deal to add to the care provided by GPs.

There are two main areas where nurses operate better than doctors, these being in areas of care that can be managed by protocols and with conditions which require regular follow-up.

Conditions managed by protocols

It has been recognised for years that nurses are much better than their *prima donnas* GP counterparts at following and completing protocols in the management of conditions such as hypertension, diabetes, etc. Doctors seem incapable of systematically sticking to the instructions they have devised themselves, let alone those introduced by another member of their team. We are not good at data entry in pre-agreed electronic slots. It is as if our greater knowledge allows us to over-ride generally accepted norms for good medical care and attention to the detail around data recording.

Nurses, on the other hand, are prepared to meticulously follow care plans, asking all the appropriate questions when prompted by a template. In this way, data collection is much more likely to be complete and stored in the appropriate place.

This attention to detail spills over into the follow-up of chronic diseases. A GP normally uses his appointment system as a follow-up system; nurses, on the other hand, recognise the difference and are frequently prepared to trawl through patients' records in order to ensure that the Practice's audit figures are more than acceptable.

Any condition that required long-term follow-up may be reduced to a protocol and given to a suitable trained nurse to manage and follow-up. The list opposite details what is currently being undertaken by our nurses.

> I don't do blood pressure any longer! This is managed almost exclusively by our nurses, but our Practice audit figures have never been better. I would suggest that there was a moral here somewhere!

The Practice's asthmatic patients have never been better managed – without any real input from me! I am deskilled. I know how to use a nebuliser with the smaller dose of Salbutamol and oral steroids in the acute situation, but as for step one, two and three – oh, and four – I know little. (Mark you, I am sure I could re-learn this information fairly quickly if I ever changed Practices.)

Minor ailments

Another thing that nurses can do is to help out with minor ailments.

The history of this development goes back some years when it was noted that doctors were quite content to see a surgery of patients, but when a couple of 'extras' with sore throats or ears were added to the end of his list, it was felt irksome. After due training in terms of the diseases and their associated medical treatments, a notice was placed on the wall of our surgery advising patients that a nurse was available to see patients who were suffering from any of 13 common conditions.

It was made clear to our receptionists that patients should not be offered appointments at the Minor Ailment Clinic because there were no appointments with the doctor, but rather as an alternative choice to a medical consultation.

After our nurse saw the patients and confirmed that he or she was in fact suffering from one of the qualifying conditions, then she would write a prescription and bring it to the GP for signature, after a discussion of the case.

This development has proved most popular, to such a degree that nurses Minor Ailment Clinics times have been regularly increased. Her holistic approach ensures that her appointments are preferentially requested to the doctors' who frequently have free appointments when nurses are completely booked!

The Minor Ailment Clinic

- The Minor Ailment Clinic has been set up to give patients the opportunity to see a nurse for common medical conditions, including the following:
  - Throat infections
  - Ear infections
  - Simple chest infections
  - Childhood rashes
  - Cystitis
  - Vaginitis and vaginal discharge
  - Insect bites and stings
  - Other simple medical matters
- Sister will liaise with your doctor if necessary, or refer you to him if your problem appears more complicated than first thought

Practice care assistant

Over the course of a week, one of our treatment room nurses ran a PDSA study to measure how many of the tasks she undertook required a nursing degree. Over the period studied, it was felt that only 46% made use of her qualification! I believe if this cycle were to be repeated, the percentage would be much higher.

Work that care assistants can do as well as nurses

- Treatment room nursing tasks
  - Venepuncture, ECGs, audiometry, BP reading, chaperoning
- Clinic nursing tasks
  - Clinical audit – asthma, diabetes, hypertension, IHD,
  - Trawling 'overdue' patients
  - Spirometry, prior to clinic
  - Equipment checks
  - Stock control

When presenting this information, I often break off to ask my audience how much they pay their chaperones? After a moment's thought their bewilderment at the question – for it's not something about many doctors think – they understand what I'm getting at. We often use our most expensive nursing colleague to perform this fairly mindless task – sometimes at F, G or even H Grade salary! This is not exactly working to the limits of our skills!

One remembers with considerable interest what happened on Friday afternoon in hospital wards: the Ward Sister would lock herself away in the cupboard to stock take! – the most expensive nursing professional in the ward counting medical and nursing cans of beans! The supermarkets call it shelf stacking.

At least our spirometers get checked regularly now; patients who have failed their follow-up are identified and contacted; we can refer patients to the treatment room which is no longer blocked by patients having ECGs and blood tests; patients do not have to wait two weeks for an audiogram; and our nurse who runs the Chest Clinic can see more patients as our care assistant provides her with the results of the spirometry she has previously performed.

When we advertised for our care assistant, we had a favourable response from the local community – indeed some people working some distance away thought the job sounded interesting. We were happy that we could appoint a good candidate.

Just before we drew up the short list, one of our more retiring receptionists approached me and said, "Dr Warrender, can I apply for the care assistant's job?" This was not quite what I had had in mind. I was looking for someone from outside, and anyway, the young lady in question was a Receptionist! I needed her where she was.

"Of, course, you can!" I heard myself say. "Fill in an application form and you'll be treated the same as everyone else" – that would be my let out clause.

On the day, there was no doubt that this young lady was the best candidate and was appointed to the job – and I have the further expense of advertising for another receptionist!

It has been a pleasure to watch the transformation in the individual we selected. Her popularity with staff and patients alike has ensured her role has been an unqualified success. As a Practice, we can point to this as an example of putting the Practice values into practice, patients, staff and efficiency! This is staff development. She is now seen as a member of the clinical staff (with an appropriate uniform) and no longer has to come in on a Saturday morning to act as receptionist – additionally she is pretty good at booking her own clinic appointments on the computer!

It has been noticed more than once that when a GP partner goes on annual leave, the two that remain can cope quite well. When the nurses who run the Chronic Disease Management Clinic go on holiday, they, too, simply cancel their clinics. When the treatment room nurses go off, we begin to notice that it's not so easy to get things done, as this commonly used, shared resource begins to get busy. But it is loss of our care assistant, however, that we really fear! For when she is not working, all the work that she has taken out of the system creeps back in, slowing it up as it goes. Everything takes longer: blood tests and other investigations are slower so that patient's problems are not sorted out as quickly and the beginnings of a dreaded backlog starts.

Shifting from the constraint

What all this demonstrates is the value of the principle that where queues and delays develop, work should be shifted from the constraint and managed in another way, often by someone else.

Constraint theory would indicate that in any system where there are a series of steps, the main constraint should be identified. This is usually fairly easy to find, in that it is preceded by a queue, pile of papers or a delay of some kind.

Having identified the major constraint, work to satisfy that constraint with everything needed to make the process more efficient, working it to its maximum capacity.

Demand management or workload shifts

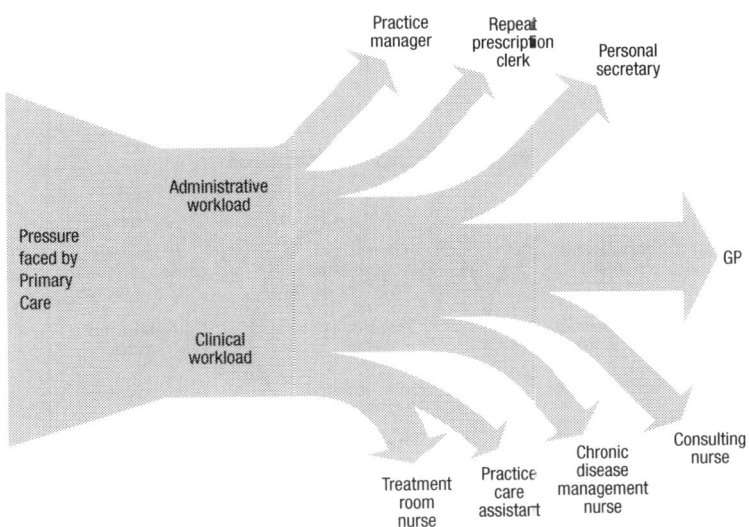

33

If this does not relieve the delay, then divert excess work to other parts of the system.

When the original delays have been shifted, re-examine the system to identify the next constraint. This search and examination must be a continuous activity, for as we will see later, solutions share shelf-life dates with supermarkets! What is a solution today may become a problem tomorrow.

Blood pressure management in Mercheford House

The diagram below shows the organisation behind our Practice hypertension protocol, and demonstrated the way that work may be distributed to ensure that all staff are working to the limits of their knowledge, skill and professional qualifications.

- It is important to realise that everybody in a Practice should have knowledge of clinical protocols, for I have not yet found one that does not affect every department in a Practice. This shared knowledge reduces duplication with respect to delivering on the planned care.
- In the case of blood pressure care, it is important that our receptionists understand that doctors do not 'do blood pressure' any longer, and that we will simply refer patients to the nurse-led BP Clinic. This could mean a wasted appointment that could have been used to see a patient on the day he or she chose!
- Thus, no matter from which source a patient with suspected hypertension has been referred, he or she should visit the BP Clinic on at least four occasions. According to the Protocol,

Hypertension cycles – 3

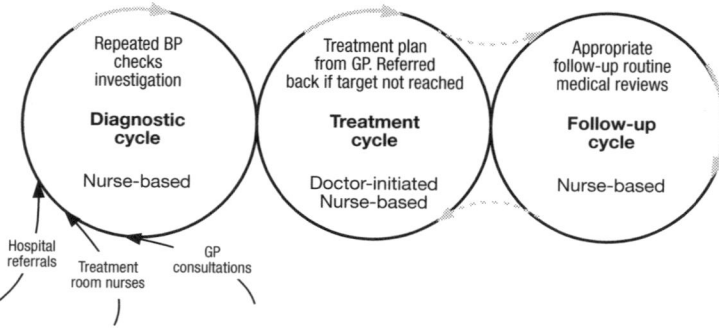

two BP readings are taken at each occasion. If the patient is found to be hypertensive after the second reading, pre-agreed blood tests are taken, and an ECG is performed. It is only at this stage, when a diagnosis has been truly made that the patient is referred to the GP. The nurse has acted to the limit of her skill, knowledge and professional qualifications.

- At the consultation, the GP has the series of BP readings to confirm the diagnosis; he has the blood results and ECG to help identify target organ involvement; he has the patient on whom he can perform a physical examination, thus having all the information necessary to agree a treatment plan with the patient.

- He can go on to explain his choice of, perhaps, three drugs, explaining their mode of action and possible side effects, before suggesting that the patient should start with the first. After three or four weeks, he or she should make an appointment with the nurse to have his or her BP measured.

> "If your blood pressure is normal when sister sees you next at the Blood Pressure Clinic in 3–4 weeks time, good and well; she will tell you when to come back to the clinic for follow-up. If your BP has not reached the target value I have written here in your card, she will speak to me and I will leave a prescription for the second drug about which we spoke. You should take this ALONG WITH the first one, and see sister three to four weeks later. If your BP is still not down to the target value, she will again inform me, and I will leave another prescription for the third drug about which we spoke, and you should see her in three to four weeks after that. At any time, if your BP is found to be above your target value on two consecutive occasions she will send you back to see me."

- Patients then pass into a follow-up cycle which means that their blood pressure is monitored regularly, according to the current protocol, and are referred back to the doctor every 2 years for a physical check.

In this scenario, each member of staff is doing what only what he or she needs to do. We are working to the limits of our knowledge, skill, professional qualifications and training to the patient's best advantage. A doctor may only be involved once every two years.

This example shows what may be done using tight protocols, efficient systems and suitably trained staff and can be transferred to conditions other than hypertension.

Whole Practice Involvement

Another principle that this blood pressure management system exemplifies is that of Whole Practice Involvement. The argument

Whole Practice Involvement

- To deal with the piles of work presented to your Practice, involve all staff to the limits of their:
  - Knowledge
  - Skill
  - Ability to learn
- Shifting specific tasks between staff can create **clinical space**

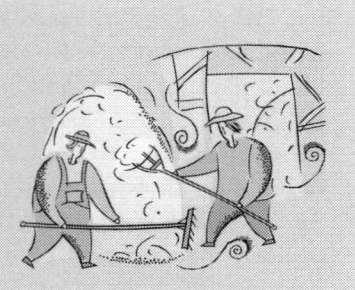

here is that everybody, but everybody, who works in a General Practice is involved in the care of the registered patients. Doctors and nurses obviously fall into this category, but it is a fact well known to many receptionists and secretaries that certain patients chose their time to come to the surgery – knowing that the doctors and nurses will not be present in order to speak with the receptionist! Care, it must be remembered, involves the improvement of the lot of another. Receptionists and secretaries often do this by a kind word or sympathetic approach. A good telephone manner is often the first thing that marks a patient's improvement – especially when it says, "And when would you like to see Doctor?"

We should respect this involvement in care – while at the same time recognising the need for confidentiality which is paramount. We should enable our staff; we should encourage them and develop their confidence. This means that a static state can never be reached, for such would be true only if a limit to their ability to learn new knowledge or skills has been reached. It is often through the development of one member of staff that another may take up the offer of training after previously declining the opportunity.

This then can create an ever-changing situation where the shift of work between ALL the care professionals who work in a surgery (or hospital) can result in the creation of clinical space.

Hay comes in stacks and bales; Practice work can be thought of in terms of hay. Using one metaphor, the work exists as a large pile in the centre, and staff are encouraged to do the tasks that can be most efficiently and appropriately done by them; the imagery of bales of hay, however, would represent pre-grouped tasks all of which might or might not be suited to an individual, over which an individual exerts an exclusive control or with the delivery of which a single individual struggles.

Let me pose a conundrum. How did the purchase of a new carpet cleaner result in the creation of more appointments with a GP?

This is mine and I'm not moving!

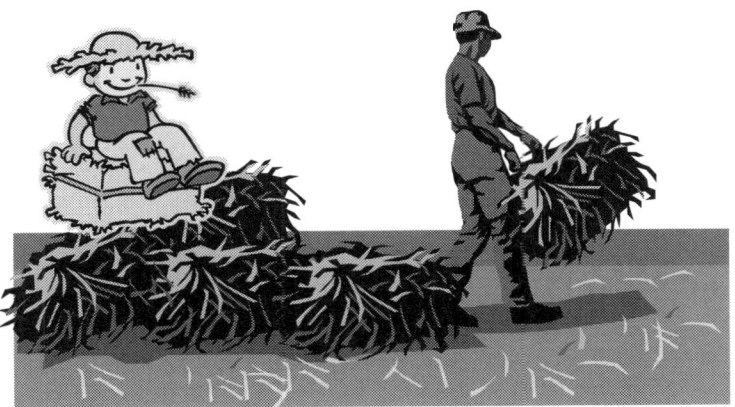

The story goes that a practice moved into its own premises about 12 years previously. The partners had the place renovated and were delighted by the results. In their excitement, the fact that only their consulting rooms and the waiting room were carpeted did not seem to worry anyone. A suitable carpet cleaner was purchased. This was moved between the three rooms – and upstairs twice a week.

The partnership grew, and a third doctor joined. The work of the Practice mushroomed, and an extension slightly larger than the footprint of the original building was added. The flooring was reconsidered, and all the new offices and clinic rooms were carpeted – but the same twelve-year-old carpet cleaner, with its daily application of cellotape to the broken plastic casing, was faithfully used.

One evening, one of the cleaners said to one of the GPs, "This is terrible. You'll need to do something about this carpet cleaner!"

"What do you mean?" he asked as she re-plugged the electric lead into one of the wall mounted sockets, and stuck on another piece of cellotape to keep the appliance together.

"Do you know! I spend nearly three quarters of an hour every night hoovering this place. The lead is so short. I have to keep replacing it when I accidentally pull it out of the socket. The attachments don't work, and I have to keep sticking the thing together. If you got me a new carpet cleaner with one of those long extension cables, I could plug it in once to do all this side of the building, and once when I came to the other." She wondered if she had gone too far. "And it would keep your cellotape bill down!"

He thought for a moment. "What kind of carpet cleaner would you like?"

She named her make and model, thinking to herself, "Yes. I won't hold my breath!"

A week passed before she opened the cleaning cupboard door to find her new carpet cleaner with its long extension cable.

A further week passed before their shifts coincided again.

"How are you doing with the new carpet cleaner?"

"It's great! I can whiz round the place in half the time. It's fab!"

"Half the time...", thought the doctor – who might have been Scottish. "Half the time..." he repeated. "That means you've saved about 20 minutes, if my memory serves me correctly. Listen, I'd like you to do some receptionists work."

"What do you mean? I'm the cleaner. I can't come in during surgery hours."

"No, no. That's not what I mean", the doctor explained. "What I would like you to do is to check that the clinic rooms and the doctor's consulting rooms have supplies of MSU bottles, and blood forms and things like that. I'll get one of the receptionists to show you."

"Oh, that's all right. I thought you meant...'

"No, no. I'll speak to Mary in the morning," said the doctor as he left.

In the morning, he spoke with Mary, the senior receptionist. "Mary, you know how you have made life a bit easier for the patients and the receptionists by making sure the doctors have supplies of MSU and FOB containers?"

"Yes. That was a good idea for it helps keep down the queues at reception. Oh, you mean there has been a problem?"

"No," the doctor interjected quickly. "No. The system has worked well since you took it over. Remember that I know you are the only completer-finisher in the building! No, what I'd like is for you to show Jenny what you do, and leave it to her – though you may want to check now and again that things are still up to your standard!"

"OK. I see what you mean. I'll speak to her tonight. I should see her before I leave"

"Excellent," the doctor murmured as he half turned to go. "By the way, how do you fancy..."

"I thought there would be trade off! I was wondering when you would get to it!" she joked.

"Well, I was thinking, how do you fancy doing some more clinical work that the nurses are doing just now?" The doctor started, only to be interrupted by Mary.

"Clinical work?" she inquired. "Clinical work? You have always said that the reception area was not the place for clinical work. You don't even want us to look into patient records for results of smears in front of patients!" She had obviously remembered one of the more recent clinical governance half-days.

"No, no. That's not what I mean. You know how Liz produces lists of patients who have not come for their asthma and blood

Creation of clinical space

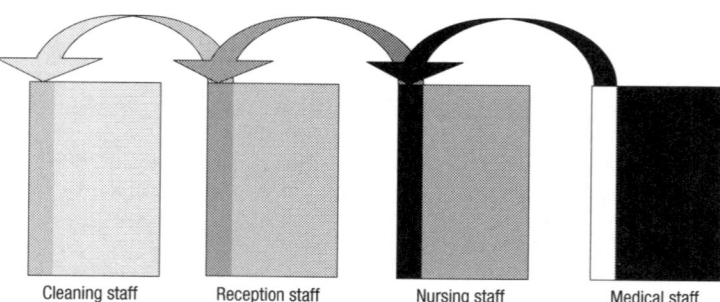

| Cleaning staff | Reception staff | Nursing staff | Medical staff |

pressure checks? What I'd like is for you to take responsibility for contacting these patients, either by phone on by letter, making sure that they have appointment at the clinics."

"Oh, *that* kind of clinical work! Yes, I'd like that. I could do it over lunch time when the surgery is closed – when I normally check the rooms....". The doctor saw the penny drop in the receptionist's mind. "I see what you're doing! You're moving work round again, like you did last time. I was wondering when you would have you next brainwave," she teased.

"Nothing to do with me!" he said as he beat a hasty retreat. "It's Jenny's fault for asking for a new carpet cleaner!"

"What's a new carpet cleaner got to do with it? I don't know what a new carpet cleaner has got to do with anything," puzzled Mary as she locked up that night.

It was the following afternoon that he bumped into his Lead Nurse. "Liz," he tried to call innocently. "Have you got a second?"

"I was wondering when you were going to get round to speaking to me! I've had Mary on to me for some lists of BP patients? What's going on?"

"It's getting to be a long story, but I thought I could move some paperwork away from you. I know how you like lists and letters and envelopes, and all that! What I had thought was that if you were to sub-contract out the recalling of patients – not the recall – simply the sending for the patients you have selected, it would save you time. You could do some more clinical work – you might be able to see another couple of minor ailment patients. You mentioned at the last Practice meeting things were getting busy again."

"Oh, I see, but I wish you had mentioned it to me first. I had no idea what Mary was on about. She must have thought I was simple."

"No, I doubt that, Liz. More like she recognised I was shifting work around again. Anyway I'll grovel to her as well as you. But at least I can also tell her about your two new Minor Ailment Clinic appointments, which will free me up to see a couple of more patients in the day they want to be seen. Thanks, Liz. You're a wonderful woman!"

Liz made an odd noise that might have represented speech as she laughed and returned to Clinic Room 1.

Late bottleneck in Mercheford House

Even though patients get into Mercheford House and see the appropriate carer, things can still go wrong. Patients can fall foul of the effects of a less than efficient system.

In order to have early intelligence as to where queues are developing, we have arranged for our staff to provide us with weekly measures of pressure in our various departments.

Using the measure of the third available appointment, data are presented with respect to the areas listed opposite.

Weekly clinic monitoring: (third available appointment)

- Investigations
  - Bloods and ECGs
- Treatment room appointments
- Chronic Disease Management Clinics
  - Asthma, blood pressure, CHD, cervical smear, chest, diabetes, pill
- Future doctors' appointments over the next four weeks

It was interesting that on one occasion, there appeared to be a delay of several weeks for patients to be seen at our nurse-led Diabetic Clinic, while there were unused appointments at the Hypertensive and Ischaemic Heart Disease Clinics. This was a bit silly when the same nurses ran all three clinics.

The problem was quickly solved by re-badging a couple of BP and IHD clinics as Diabetic Clinics and things got back into balance.

Other ideas for reducing bottlenecks

Primary care examples of late bottlenecks solutions

- Use of care assistant
  - Blood tests done on the day
  - Instant chaperoning
- Recall management as distinct to the appointment system
- Use (and refreshing) of Practice protocols
- Use of care templates in the Practice
- Use of telephones and secretaries

Listed opposite are other simple concepts and ideas that we have found useful in keeping the flow of patient care through Mercheford House running smoothly.

- Having a care assistant who is able to perform blood tests on the same day as the consultation saves our more elderly patients coming up for a plurality of visits while they are being investigated. This not only is good for our patients, but it saves on administrative time which can be translated into clinical time.

One habit – of which I am not particularly proud – was that of asking female patients to make a further appointment with the treatment room nurse and myself at a later date when they presented with a gynaecological complaint. These were in fact double appointments to allow for the delay that either the nurse or the doctor was experiencing on the day.

Basically, this meant that most gynaecological problems, however simple or complex, took up to five appointments. Now, we simply ask the care assistant, armed with her case containing all the necessary instruments, etc., to come through to our consulting rooms where the patient's problems can be dealt with at a single visit.

Four appointments are saved for patients who want to see the doctor of their choice on the day of their choice – and our receptionists are spared the tricky problem of trying to fit in 'double appointment with doctor and nurse'.

- We have developed the concept that recall management is intrinsically different to the running of an appointment system. Doctors are fairly good at knowing and measuring what they do; we are not as good as knowing what we **do not** do. It has been claimed that by using our appointment system as a recall system, we can kill two birds with the one stone. This is not really true:

- We are not always sure our patients have made a follow-up appointment
- We do not always act on the fact that our patients have not attended [DNA'd]

Having a system dedicated to identifying patients who have conditions that need to be tracked and follow-up up means that their visits may be fed into a more flexible appointment system that is not clogged up with an extensive backlog. Our hospital colleagues would benefit from understanding the increased flexibility this confers.

- Reference has already been made to the need for refreshing clinical protocols, but the point bears repeating, for it does offer scope to reduce work load.

- It greatly saves the overall work performed in a Practice if all clinicians record clinical information in the same way.

The story goes that in one Practice, some of the GPs were better at transferring work to their IHD nursing lead than others. The other doctors saw her as being overloaded and tried to spare her by reviewing IHD patients themselves in surgery.

Those doctors who had managed to struggle with their consciences to transfer patients across to the Nurses Clinic felt guilty that they were getting home on time and had heard no complaints from the nurse.

All was made clear when the annual external audit was run. The nurse started pulling out her hair when she saw the clinic's relatively low figures. This in turn led to a bolus of work she and her team could have done without. During the trawl of the patient records, it became clear that although the doctors who had been trying to spare her work had been asking the appropriate question of the patients, they had either not recorded the information, or recorded in it in places where external search programs had not been instructed to look.

Many hours, records and patients later, the nurse managed to regain her high audit position.

The moral of the story is simply this: if doctors are going to compete with nurses in areas in which nurses undoubtedly do better, they have got to learn how to use templates and stick to protocols. If, on the other hand, they leave their nursing colleagues to do what they do well, they may enjoy being de-skilled in yet another area!

- In our Practice the doctors are fortunate enough to have individual secretaries. This creates the opportunity for these wonderful colleagues to act as direct and consistent intermediaries between GP, patients and the outside world. Perhaps this is one reason why we have not gone down the potentially valuable road of nurse triage – we may be using our secretaries in a similar way. Also, by operating an Advanced Access system, we know we can cope with the clinical workload generated by our patients. What we do not know, but will be investigating, is whether our patients would prefer increased phone contact rather than a physical appointment.

- The two pictures set out below represent system improvements initiated by my secretary. They follow the improvement principle of providing all that is necessary to make a decision or complete an action at a single point in time

Move steps closer together

Identify and manage constraints

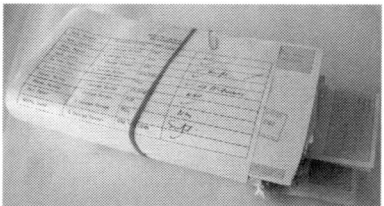

Move steps closer together

Identify and manage constraints

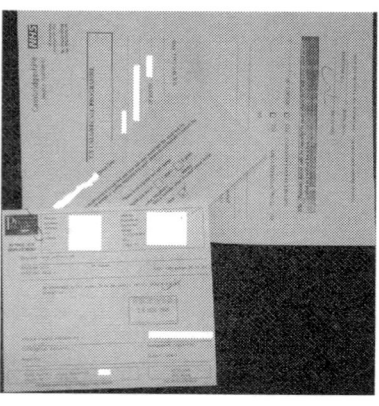

– **Dealing with investigation reports**

What often happened in the Practice was that when the results came through, they were presented to the doctor who checked through them, annotating each form and requesting the notes of patients whose results required to be actioned. Some time later – perhaps even a day or two, depending whether he was on a day off or so – he would get the notes and make a decision. This in turn might take another 24 hours to be completed by the secretary

In the new system, our secretaries make a list of the patients whose investigations are to hand, with room for comment and action points. Enclosed are the notes of patients whose medical envelopes I am likely to want, i.e. those with abnormal results. This means that at a single sitting, I have all that is required to complete the whole exercise with minimal delay.

– A second example of this principle might be the way the smear results are processed. On this occasion, I am presented with the original smear result, the note to inform the patient of the result and the letter to the HA to remove the patient's name from its recall list if she has not reached that point.

In the past, several hand-offs and delays would have been encountered and patients not always removed from the recall system.

Late system constraints:

Poor parcel exit

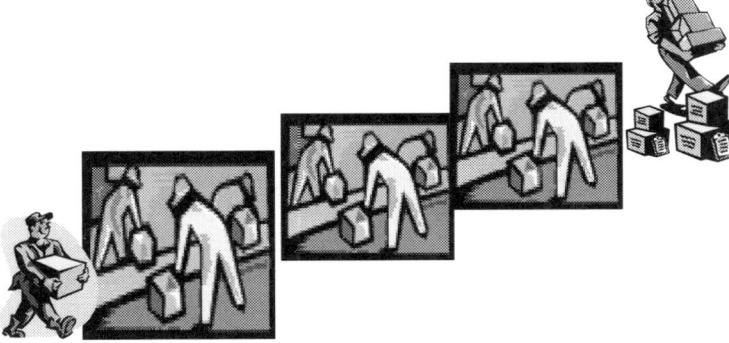

Poor patient exit

In the last part of this chapter, I should like to describe how doctors or nurses can make matters difficult for our reception colleagues. With a little bit of forethought, we could reduce their workload to allow them time for more clinical tasks that would in turn create more clinical space in which GPs could see patients on the day they wished to be seen.

It would make sense to attempt to keep the numbers of patients presenting at the reception desk to a minimum. This would include deciding where patients should pick up urine sample bottles, make transport bookings, ask for repeat prescriptions, investigation results and other pseudo-clinical issues. By diverting away from the constraint of the reception area, we make it easier for our staff to do their job quietly and efficiently.

Patients who are unsure of their next appointment can create a lot of unnecessary work. Although doctors and nurses do try to make it clear to patients when they should return and with whom they should make their next appointment, the anxiety of the consultation often ensures that this has been forgotten by the time the patient reaches the receptionist.

The use of a form completed by the doctor or nurse and given to the patient simplifies matters tremendously, and reduces work at the front desk. An example of one used in Mercheford House is shown opposite.

One of the most certain ways to waste receptionists' time is to pay them to make appointments (with the thought that that often entails), then pay the

Appointment slip

Mercheford House Appointment Slip

If you have been asked to make an appointment within the next four weeks, please contact one of our receptionists and she will complete the date and time on this appointment slip.

If your appointment is more than 4 weeks away, our reception staff will give you an approximate date for your appointment which you should confirm nearer the time.

Appointment details

Date:			Time:				
GP/Clinic	Days	Wks	Month	S	A	R	
TSW/EJW/DAH							
Joint appointments							
T/R	C/A						

How to make it even more difficult for receptionists!

- Do not tell them when you are giving an important meeting or presentation
- Keep your annual leave a secret
- Have them cancel surgeries and clinics – then have them re-make the same appointments
- Do not speak to them
- Keep interrupting them by telephone
- Don't tell them that you're glad you employed them – till they leave!

same staff to cancel these appointments, only to ask them to make them again on another day! It transforms what might be a rewarding occupation into something that is not always looked forward to on Monday mornings!

The important point to make here is that it is difficult to argue for more money from the Primary Care Organisations if we waste what we already have been given in ways similar to this.

Some other ways to make receptionist's life less than perfect are set out above.

In summary

In this chapter I have tried to anchor the principle of Advanced Access in Practice culture, organisation and systems. It is only by so doing that these initial ideas are sustainable.

- Advanced Access should not be attempted in the absence of a stable Practice where there is no shared vision. Whole Practice involvement is required.
- In order to get that involvement, staff must feel valued, and their contribution to the broader aspects of patient care acknowledged and respected. Staff must want to take part in the delivery of the vision and values of the Practice.
- Nurses are a main stay of Advanced Access. They must be willing and able to take on the important role of delivering the Practice's Chronic Disease Management Programme. Without them, such access cannot be brought about. Allowing them to undertake this role by delegating work they do not have to do to others is equally important. As a means of expanding this argument, the Practice must have the appropriate mix of skill, knowledge and staff to deliver its total care agenda.
- Patients must be helped to understand our new ways of working, and become as willing to see other members of the Practice team as their regular GP. This shift can only be

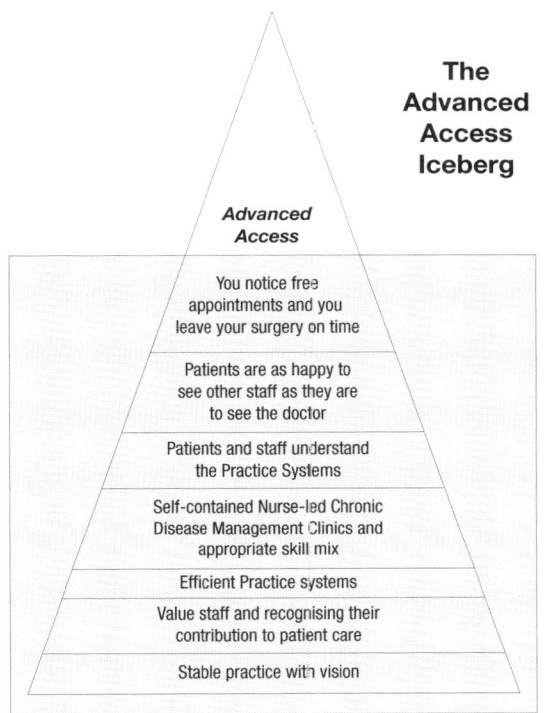

The Advanced Access Iceberg

Advanced Access

You notice free appointments and you leave your surgery on time
Patients are as happy to see other staff as they are to see the doctor
Patients and staff understand the Practice Systems
Self-contained Nurse-led Chronic Disease Management Clinics and appropriate skill mix
Efficient Practice systems
Value staff and recognising their contribution to patient care
Stable practice with vision

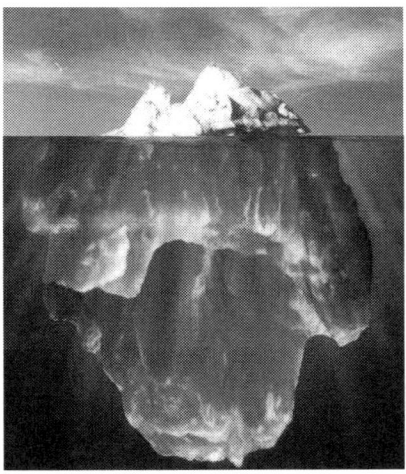

The highly visible achievement of *'seeing patients on the day of their choice'* or *'doing today's work today'*, is only possible when it is supported by less visible but more important culture, organisation and systems that must pre-exist within the Practice

brought about by their doctors. Patients will understand this by what the doctor says as well as how their doctors are seen to respect their colleagues to whom their patient care is being transferred.

- It is time to think about committing to Advanced Access when doctors notice substantial changes and benefit to their work/life balance.
- Finally, we will have to bear in mind that the visible part of the iceberg in the picture above would never appear and stay above the surface of the sea were it not for another seven eighths of mass underwater! So it is with Advanced Access.

Advanced Access is eminently 'do-able' but it does require a fundamental re-think of what we currently do. It is fun; it brings back an excitement about our work.

The next chapter will describe some pointers you may wish to consider in planning its implementation.

Chapter 3

Change

Change and how to do it

Before making comment about making change in a General Practice, I should like to make a few comments related to its place in care delivery.

As long as we have General Practice as we currently know it, with doctors having independent contractor status delivering care to a registered patient base, General Practice will be the unit through which primary care will be provided. Neither Strategic Health Authorities nor Primary Care Organisations can undertake that role.

This being the case, everybody in the Practice delivers care, and has the right to be involved in care delivery. Care, as has been defined elsewhere in this book is the improving the lot of another. This extends the function of care from the purely clinical – delivered by doctors and nurses – to that provided by each and every member of the Practice Team.

Not all care has been traditionally noticed or valued. Care usually starts when a patient rings up for an appointment, and continues when a secretary is asked about the results of blood tests and the like. The way the communication is conducted has a direct effect on the outcome. Care continues when patients sit in a quiet and clean waiting area that is not over-crowded with delayed patients. This means that everybody in the team has the right to become involved in care re-design and the associated changes that it involves. In fact it is likely that the changes will only be maximally effective if all those involved in the various processes are involved in the changes.

Solutions that have been developed in other situations or Practices are unlikely to work as well as they did in the Practice in which they were developed. Answers are not usually transferable.

The idea here is that while the principles on which the changes are based are common to all, and the final product (in this care, Advanced Access) is shared by all, the methods or means chosen

> **Primary assumptions**
>
> - The practice is the unit of Primary Care delivery
> - Care is delivered by everybody in the practice
> - Everybody has the right to be involved
> - Nurses will save the NHS
> - Imported solutions unlikely to work
> - Understanding the need for change
> - Individuals create change – it's up to you!
> - Change works better when everybody concerned is involved in the changes
> - The importance of anticipating change

to deliver the final product or vision must, of necessity be home grown – and growth, as we all know, takes time.

This is why spread of good practice has proved so difficult and elusive; while the principle of the wheel should not be invented at each and every site, the way the wheel is used to produce vehicular movement must be situation specific – even though the final product (the vehicle) may be similar.

What this chapter will be at pains to stress is the need for individual Practices to 'do it their way!'

The importance of leaders

It is very unlikely successful change will take place if the need for change is not understood and shared by all concerned. This boils down to communication by the leaders of the Practice team.

The pain of change is only worthwhile if it runs true to the culture in which we operate. By this, I mean that if, as a Practice, the leaders are seen to be driven by externally set target figures or performance tables, staff will see them as such. If the changes are thought to be driven by the partner's desire for more money or simple kudos, this too will soon become evident.

If, however, the improvement being designed is consistent with the demonstrable values and culture of the Practice concerned, then there is a much better feeling, and the changes are much more likely to be implemented and sustained. Mercheford House values of *Patients, Staff and Efficiency* have gone a long way to aid the change process.

It should be understood that individuals, not organisations initiate change; organisations effect change, but only after they have been brought to it by individuals. Change associated with improvement usually starts with someone having an idea, a notion around doing things differently, being smarter. This can happen equally well in the privacy of a bath or in a more public group meeting! It is the sharing of the bright idea with others that takes the idea on its way to implementation. While a committee may be needed to knock the wall down to make the changes to the Practice architecture, it may well have been the new receptionist's idea that started it all off.

Unless these fleeting notions are shared, recorded and evaluated, the idea may be lost for ever, or at least till someone else has the same thought. If the idea is strangled at birth by a more senior member of staff with whom it is initially shared, not only does it evaporate, but the way in which it is handled may well ensure that no idea is shared by the individual in the future. Leaders must listen as well as speak and do.

It may seem counter-productive and time-wasting to involve all staff in the making of big decisions around change, but it is usually folly to attempt to do so without their knowledge and help. Not only is ownership of an idea important, but staff who work in specific areas usually know more about that area than the partners. They will be quick to comment on the feasibility of any change.

This concept has been developed by Goldratt[1] who advocates a Socratic approach to gaining staff involvement. By asking questions of our staff and helping them to develop their own ideas, they can give birth to the idea personally – the emotional involvement being much stronger that the emotion of fear that usually meets the thought of change.

This method of developing a change improvement agenda has certainly been found to work in Mercheford House, where, by the end of the meetings, ideas have progressed far beyond our original objectives or hopes.

Solutions that change have time limitations and restrictions. Ideas around the constancy of change must be developed within every Practice, and even the good solutions need to be re-examined and updated.

The seven principles for effective change

As a format for this chapter, I should like to use (and modify) the principles of change described by Nadlar & Hibino[2] as they address the issues faced by General Practice so well.

1 The uniqueness principle

This simply states that what works in one Practice may not necessarily work in another – or it will produce even better results. Imported solutions are unlikely to be successful as they were developed in a unique combination of circumstances in terms of:

- Staff, their personalities, knowledge and skills
- Facilities, geography and Practice layout
- The precise nature of the common problem being examined and the local circumstances

[1] *Theory of Constraints*, 1990. Eliyahu M. Goldratt. North River Press.

[2] *Breakthrough Thinking*, 1994. Gerald Nadlar and Sozo Hibino. Prima Publishing.

Seven principles of effective change

1. The uniqueness principle
2. The purposes principle
3. The solution-after-next principle
4. The systems principle
5. The limited information collection principle
6. The people design principle
7. The betterment timeline principle

The uniqueness principle

- No two situations are alike

- Each problem is embedded in a unique array of related problems – identify all your peculiarities and local circumstances

- The solution to a problem in one organisation will differ in some way from the solution to a similar problem in another organisation

All these ensure that no two situations are alike, although they may appear to address the same issues. This means the solutions, must, of necessity be different. In other words, the **product** – seeing patients on the day of their choice – may be shared; the **principles** are common – to be used in all situations; but the **processes** used to arrive at the end point are unique to each Practice situation.

All these individual peculiarities need to be understood in great detail before introducing changes. Once appreciated, it will be easily understood why the processes that work in one area cannot pertain to another. It is usually much quicker, having heard about the processes and solution that have been successful in another place, to go back to the principles, and to redesign NEW processes rather than to adapt these old ones from other sites.

The ubiquitous SWOT analysis[3] has a place in the planning of solutions. The strength of this approach is often weakened in that it is repeated as circumstances change. In other words, as changes are gently implemented the results of the SWOT analysis should be kept current and in date.

2   The purposes principle

In all but the very simplest situation, these are a variety of possible solutions to any particular problem. The purposes principle simply focuses the mind on deciding exactly what it is we are trying to do.

The purposes principle

- There is seldom a problem where a single solution meets all the needs

- Involve all who have a view and an interest

- Think in terms of arrays of needs

- Select the focal purpose

- Devise measures to plot progress and effectiveness

There is seldom a solution to a problem of any complexity that meets all the needs that exist, and we must have a very clear idea of precisely what it is we are trying to correct, improve or develop. We need to involve everyone in the Practice who has a view or an interest in the particular area. By discussing the problem openly and freely, it will be found that there are always an array of purposes: the receptionists see one thing as the main issue, whereas, the secretaries see another. The nurses, on the other hand, see the problem through more clinical eyes as something altogether different. What is being developed is a horizontal array of purposes.

If further thought be given to almost any situation, a vertical array is quickly developed as it become apparent that by widening the purpose, considerably greater gain or improvement might be delivered.

[3] SWOT analysis is a simple way of listing a Practice's Strengths, Weaknesses, Opportunities and Threats. Used honestly and with humour, a SWOT session can be most valuable.

At a whole staff Practice meeting, Mary reported that Mrs White, a patient of Dr Frank's has passed comment that she had not had the result of her last cervical smear. "And it was taken four weeks ago," the whole waiting room had heard.

"That was not my fault!" Fay almost shouted – she was not feeling at her best that day. "I'm sorry, but I didn't see the result. It was under that new diabetic protocol Liz gave me," she said, darting a look in the Practice manager's direction.

"It was partly my fault. I was a bit slow in getting it through to you," said Dr Frank, trying to swallow his crisps.

"Why do the doctors need to see the results of smears, anyway?" asked Karen. "Anyone can see that a normal smear is a normal smear!"

"Usually that's true, but medico-legally I think we should see the results before they go to patients." Dr James was always the most cautious among the three doctors. "What I do…"

"But that's another point!" burst in Jenny, the Practice Manager. "Why do we have three systems in this place? Why can we not have one system, like the BP protocol – where everybody knows what everybody else does? Sorry." She flushed a little and turned to Dr James, "I didn't mean to interrupt you mid-sentence, but that was one of the common complaints – well perhaps that's too strong a word – comments at the staff appraisals. Each of you has your own different ways of working. It wastes so much time, running three parallel systems. Why can we not have one system for the whole Practice?"

There was a few seconds silence as the pennies dropped. The quiet voice of Debbie, Dr Sam's secretary commented, "If you are thinking about that, what about including the blood results. It's the same thing. Results have got to be properly checked and patients informed of the results. Why can't we have a single system for dealing with them?" She hoped Dr Sam had not thought she had spoken out of turn.

Dr Sam, ever the empathetic one, crashed in. "She's right. That was one of the things I noted when I joined the Practice: we all work differently. It must be difficult for the staff to remember what to do when." Debbie glanced at Karen, Dr Frank's secretary, remembering the conversation they had had about ordering patient transport; both did it in entirely different ways.

"What's the problem with the path results?" quizzed the Practice Manager. "Nobody has raised it as an issue before.' She turned to Dr Frank. "Can we spend 10 minutes looking at this? I'm not sure, but there might be some common themes."

"No probs." was the abbreviated reply.

Jenny stood up, wiped the white board clean, found a marker pen that worked and launched into one of her 'sessions'. "For the next five minutes, I want you to brainstorm the issues around path reports."

"I never know what to say. It's difficult being at the front desk when patients ask for their results. They think that because you are at reception, you know everything. We are the first people they see when they come into the surgery." The young receptionist looked round at Mary her senior. Perhaps she had been too quick, but Mary nodded in agreement. It was OK.

"My problem," Mary added, "is that patients seem to phone for results at our busiest times. I really find it difficult to know whether to be checking patients in, looking out notes, or contacting the secretaries for results."

"But should you be giving out results?" asked Dr James. "People may overhear you, and I do not think you should be seen to have access to the notes in the reception area in view of the patients. Saturdays and after 4.30 p.m. is different as the secretaries are usually away by that time."

"I think it should be the secretaries that deal with results," reasoned the Practice nurse. They are the ones who know most about the patients – apart from the GPs, that is. I think all the results – smear results as well as path results – should go through them. If I have a query, that's who I would go to."

Debbie, Dr Sam's Secretary had been trying to get a word in for a while. "Why don't we just go paperless, and get all the results to go directly into the computer without anybody seeing them. If a patient phoned up, then anyone could give them their results."

"It's not as easy as that. If I have to deal with the results, then I've got to know what to say. A doctor or a nurse needs to check them first." Karen was always the one that thought about practicalities. "The problem with that is that it can be up to three days delay before that patient hears after the results come to the Practice. Dr Frank asked me to check this for two weeks last month."

Dr James supported her. "But, medico-legally one of the doctors should really make sure that we see the results of all the tests we have done. I think we should keep a list of all samples that we send to the lab. That way we can be sure that everybody who has had a test gets a result from the lab in the first instance – but I've said this before, and nobody wants the work."

"Now I know that is difficult, but what would happen if I simply typed a list of everybody whose result had come back. If I then passed it to the Doctor, he could write down what he wants me to say to the patient."

"But sometimes I need to see the notes," repeated Dr. James.

"I know that," continued Karen, "but I can usually tell the abnormal results. They have 'Hi' or 'Lo' after the results. It took me a while to notice that, but it's there for everything except the bacteriology results – but that's not a problem, really. If it's abnormal, there is usually writing and 'plusses'. Anyway, Dr Frank has shown me how to check if she has given the correct antibiotics to women with cystitis. I think with a little bit of training, we could set up a system."

The Practice Manager, who had been scribing the ideas, checked her watch again. "It seems to me that there are three layers in this onion – or three layers of purpose, as we heard the other week."

"We have the inside layer of how to deal with the cervical smear reports; then the next layer – we could look at how to handle all the reports, pathology, bloods, as well as smears; and lastly we have the great outside layer that gets us paperless. I think we should go for the middle layer – what do you think?"

There was a general air of agreement. The Manager pointed to the paper flipchart near Karen. "Show us what you mean," and made to throw a marker towards her. She tossed it when Karen held out her hands to catch it.

This was the bit that Karen always hated. By the time she found a clean page on the flipchart, she was quite red in the cheeks. "I'm not very good at this, but if the results, all the results came in and were date stamped as usual." She made an arrow pointing to another square. "If each secretary was to type a list of the name and address of every patient who had a test, with their address and phone number, along with the test and a space for the doctor to write down what he wanted us to do or what to say to the patient."

"But what about the patients whose notes I need to see?" Dr James again repeated.

"The secretaries can pull the notes that are to be seen. You would have asked them to do this when you saw the results. That could save a day – sometimes two – in getting back to the patient." Nobody but Dr Frank recognised the significance of the silent glance she gave him. "Anyway," she went on, "you would have all the results, so you could ask for the notes of the ones we've missed."

"If you do that…" This was first time Fay had spoken since her defensive outburst at the beginning of the meeting "If you do that, why can't you include a note on which the patient has written her name and address when she came for a smear. Karen could make a form that had boxes the doctors could tick for the result and whether the patient needed a repeat in three or five years. That would mean that the whole problem of getting back to the patient with her result could be quite fast." Her composure had been re-captured.

"It would," added Karen, "if I attached a – that orange smear withdrawal form – the one that means that older patients and the ones who have had a hysterectomy don't need further recall. That would be really good; everything would be done in one go!"

Jenny, in true Practice Manager style, had noted Mary's gaze and her head nodding towards Dr Sam. He had been shuffling in his seat. He had four visits to do after the meeting.

"OK. Let's stop. This has been good. We seem to have got the bones of a system to deal with all investigation results coming into the Practice. If you let me have your flipchart, Karen, I'll write it up and circulate it for comment at the beginning of the week If you show the other staff how you've kept track of Dr Frank's time delays, the other two can check if this has been shortened for their own doctors. Well done, folks. That was worthwhile. Thanks. Excellent."

Nobody overheard the conversation between Drs. Frank and James as they walked down the stairs, but they seemed pleased that afternoon.

The figure overleaf demonstrates what happened at the meeting. There was a horizontal array of issues around a shared problem, that of handling the cervical smear results as seen through the eyes of the different staff members.

The issue was extended vertically to include the way ALL results were managed. This, too, produced a horizontal extension, as it affected most members of the Practice team.

Horizontal matrix of varying staff perspectives

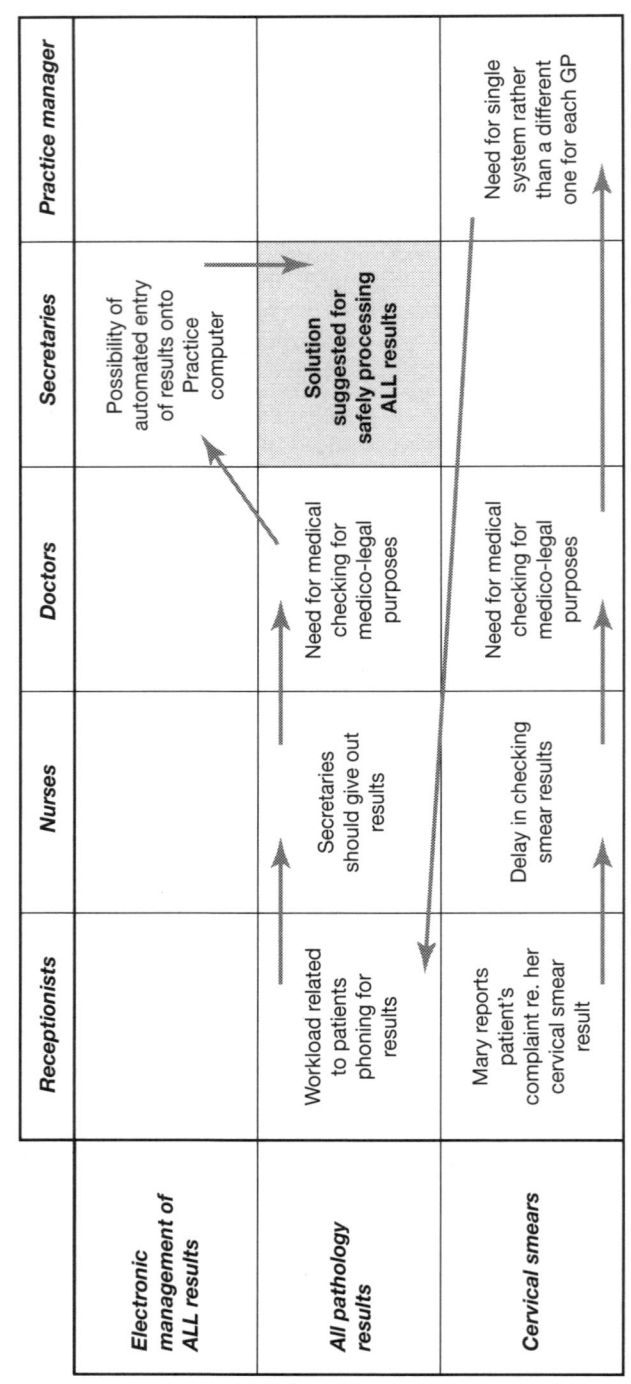

	Receptionists	Nurses	Doctors	Secretaries	Practice manager
Electronic management of ALL results				Possibility of automated entry of results onto Practice computer	
All pathology results	Workload related to patients phoning for results	Secretaries should give out results	Need for medical checking for medico-legal purposes	**Solution suggested for safely processing ALL results**	
Cervical smears	Mary reports patient's complaint re. her cervical smear result	Delay in checking smear results	Need for medical checking for medico-legal purposes		Need for single system rather than a different one for each GP

Vertical matrix of content and complexity

A further dimension was added with respect to dealing with all the results electronically and without handling paper. This scenario was a bit too far for the group.

The Practice Manager judged that the focal purpose extended further than simply dealing with smear results, but not as high as becoming paperless She was responsible for asking a colleague to lead in developing joint solutions with respect to the focal purpose, a solution that she would reduce to paper in a short and stated time frame. No wonder the two GPs were pleased!

As a general rule, when contemplating any change, a measure should be selected as an indicator of the success or otherwise of the new process. Such a measurement may be a measurable, numerical measurement such as the number of letters waiting for Doctor's signature, or the numbers of telephone calls received for investigation results; or it might be a straw pole taken one month into the changes to ensure that all the concerns raised at the meeting have been addressed, if not completely resolved.

> If you do not know where you are going or have not selected a destination, you would not know when to get off the bus!

3 The solution-after-next principle

This concept is as valuable and powerful as it is simple; it seeks to ask the question, "If you achieved what you are setting out to do, what would you want to do next?"

There are innumerable occasions when we have looked back after getting what we wanted, and said, "If only I had known, then I would have done it differently or got the bigger or different model!" This is exactly what this principle seeks to get us to think about.

Pretend you have delivered the change on which you have been working; what would you do now? This focuses the attention on as yet unseen consequences of the, as yet proposed, change.

> In the late eighties, a doctor and his wife had a discussion. She felt it imperative that the kitchen be 'done'. It has been agreed when they had moved into the house that the current kitchen furniture was far from perfect, and that it had to go as soon as the finance was available.
>
> "Has the time come," asked the wife, "when the new kitchen could be priced up?"
>
> "Yes, get a quote," unexpectedly came the reply. "It would be good to know the current prices. But you do remember that we agreed I could get a new Mercedes? Not only is the blue car falling to bits, but I would really like the new model."

The debate started, but much of it was totally irrelevant, and both knew in their heart of hearts that the money was not around – such was the influence of school fees! She really wanted to extend the kitchen to make it larger, but that meant uprooting her favourite magnolia tree – and even she knew that was not an option!

A year or so later, a strip of ground along the side of their house went up for sale. If they bought that, the kitchen could be extended without the uprooting of the tree. The matter was agreed, and the couple successfully negotiated the purchase of the land.

Not long after the extension had been built, the estimate for the new kitchen arrived by post. Further discussion!

"OK, go ahead with the kitchen, as long as I get the car within three years!"

"It's a deal," smiled a happy lady.

Five years later, after all had enjoyed the new kitchen and its furniture and its double draining sink unit that had meant the kitchen wall was two feet further from the house than the original plans had shown, the last insurance policy was about to mature. "Right, the car," thought the doctor. "But I need somewhere to keep it. I can't use the old garage." That had been long since turned into a pottery workroom. "I'm certainly not buying a Merc without some place to keep it."

As with all big decisions, the two of them discussed the matter. "What about a car port along by the side of the kitchen? You could build a roof against the fence."

"Great idea," he thought as he went out to measure up.

It was about this time disaster dawned. The new kitchen with its external pipes had not left enough room for the car port and car. "If I had only made do with a single drainer sink, or moved the whole unit to the other side as we talked about...."

The doctor still does not have his Mercedes but has learned to enjoy cooking!

This domestic scene has been replayed in many Practices up and down the land – as well as in many Hospital Trusts. 'If only we knew then what we know now....' The solution-after-next principle helps us to plan effective change – joined up change – change that leads on and connects with the future, rather than leading us up a blind alley.

The solution after-next-principle provides an opportunity to think about how we might go about finding our current solution:

- After we establish our nurse-led Diabetic Clinic, we will tackle hypertension – why not start planning NOW for the new clinic room and the training of the other nurses?
- After we switch to computer-based medical records, we will look at an electronic appointment system – perhaps you should ensure that the new clinical system you are considering purchasing has an appointment module that suits your needs and the abilities of your receptionists.

- Is the solution to your accommodation really the purchase of a second detached building? Should you not be considering relocating to another site altogether?

Using this concept routinely allows you and your staff to start visiting and visioning for the future. It starts thought about a time frame for the changes we face; it allows the development of a list of projects, and the best order in which they should be completed.

Looking to possible future solutions gives you the opportunity to look at your current initiative to ensure that they might not be tackled in other ways for greater results. It provides the opportunity to contemplate alternative futures, and goes some way to reduce the paralysis of being limited by your imagination.

The principle-after-next principle also assumes a 'shelf life' for a solution or idea. This recurrent theme will be developed later, but even the very best solutions only serve the needs and problems as they exist now. When circumstances change, so must the ideal solution.

Visioning sessions

I have been at visioning sessions that have been truly magic, and others that have been worse than disastrous! People who feel they have to be 'in control' are not always best at facilitating these groups, for the outcome, by definition is unstructured and unplanned.

It is also a challenge – which can be managed – to have people of differing intellects, rank and knowledge in the same group. It is within these groups that different views and suggestions are often made.

There are a few 'rules' for visioning session, but the main one is simply respect: respect for the individual and his or her suggestion. Ideas should not be filtered, judged or criticised as they are offered. They must be respectfully recorded on the flip chart, and only measured and judged after suggestions have stopped.

It has happened on more than one occasion that a junior in the Practice has made a comment to a more senior member of staff, only to be told, "That would not work!" Whether that be true or not, the cursive dismissal of an idea to which a junior has given birth certainly ensures that further suggestions are not readily forthcoming.

The further comment from the senior with the felt tip pen at a Practice visioning group, "I've told you before – that won't work here" is then enough to ensure silence from that moment on.

On the other hand, words do not need to be said – the quiet, critical, controlling cough from the senior partner is every bit as effective!

Rules and guidance for visioning sessions

1. Ensure that all the members of the group understand the nature of visioning
2. Make people feel that it is safe to participate
3. Check the group knows why it has met, and that they are all aware of the problem the group is trying to solve.
4. Be prepared to tackle complex issues in bite-sized chunks, relating them to the bigger picture
5. Allow some time for people to gather their thoughts
6. Encourage people to be as creative and inventive as possible, building on each others' suggestions
7. Record all ideas and suggestions as they are verbalised.
8. Have as many scribes and flipcharts as required for the group. Enlist the help of others if the existing scribes cannot write quickly enough to record all the thoughts at the time – it is unlikely they will be remembered later.
9. Questions may be asked to develop concepts, linking them to others on the chart, but...
10. Do not judge, criticise or evaluate ideas till the appropriate part of the session, and then make it plain that no idea is given preferential consideration
11. Try to get everyone to contribute, going round the group from one to the other if necessary; try to hear from the shy, silent group members.

In the same way as it was necessary to develop an array of purposes before selecting the focal purpose, an array of solutions should be generated before choosing the focal solution for the issue under debate. This may be greater or smaller than the one first thought about, but it will have the advantage of being set in a much bigger context. Your Practice people will see the direction from which you are coming, and where you would like to lead them. They will be more than happy that they have been party to the big plan, and feel they have given birth to ideas that will influence the future direction of the Practice.

4   The systems principle

Here, the message is that all actions, as well as reactions, can have unforeseen consequences. In organisational terms, a General Practice is an operational unity, a body whose parts have different functions and purposes, but which, together, delivers care to its registered patients. It is system that has been either set up or allowed to deliver the output it produces. It may not have been the GPs plan to deliver care with a 1, 3, 21 day delay, but every member of the practice works to that agenda, whether they know it or not. Every system is designed to achieve the output it produces.

When contemplating making changes to our Practice systems, remember the iceberg; seven-eighths of both are not usually seen. What is seen in a Practice is normally the outcome of the system, not the system themselves. This means, in turn, that changes – good or bad – have at least as much chance of affecting the unseen system processes as the outcomes themselves.

Taking a 'people' example, even planned improvement can alter what a member of staff does in such a way as to remove the enjoyment of the task for which he or she really came to work in the first place.

An IT example might be the unplanned pressure on a shared computer terminal that leads to difficulty in producing the repeat prescriptions in a timely fashion.

The pressure on timetabling a room or the need to alter the clinic times of another professional may be the unforeseen issues that arise from an improved care of the elderly plan.

This is one reason why it is easier to develop Practice change under the eyes of all Practice staff; each has the opportunity to understand the effects of the changes on their own little world. No single change can be seen in isolation.

For any, other than the simplest of changes, options appraisal type of analysis should be undertaken. This practice is better known to our secondary care managerial colleagues, but it is equally as vital in the smaller microcosms of General Practice, where the effects may be much more personally and keenly felt.

A matrix should be drawn up providing the opportunity to set out the effects of any particular development on the different departments within the Practice. For major undertakings, this may have to be circulated on paper to each member of staff, providing them with a chance to consider the matter in detail and formulate their thoughts. For other topics, a relaxed, open forum may be the optimal time and place.

Whatever the venue and means, the process of assessing the effects of change must be all-inclusive; all staff concerned should be involved.

This is not to say that the partnership of the Practice should abdicate the responsibility and leadership to their employees; what is being suggested is that to obtain maximal buy-in and ownership of the planned changes. This is simply the most productive way to operate. Staff must all feel themselves to be a valued part of the changes.

5   The limited information principle

It is always a matter of mild amusement to me that when planning to improve matters for the better, the first thing clinicians and managers seem to do is 'to collect the data'. They often then spend months collecting this information that serves only to make them **experts in what they already knew did not work!**

While it is obvious we need to learn what is going on under the surface of our organisation, a limit should be set when considering what does not work, spending more time and energy on devising process to make the system work better.

With this in mind, we often forget the *wisdom in the heads of people*. Receptionists who have spent years working in the same surgery, or secretaries who have become expert in what they do, often have the answers in their head to the problems the Practice may be facing as a whole. They simply have not had the opportunity to share them with anyone who can put their ideas into practice.

Prizes for the *best suggestion of the month* may seem out of place these days, but to ignore the ideas of our staff or not provide a means by which they percolate up to the collective consciousness of the Practice is a poor and dangerous action. Having read this statement, it is something we *choose* to do or not do from now on!

Having gently poked fun at data collectors, it is obvious that some data must be gathered, analysed and understood if we are to demonstrate improvement. In terms of access to Primary Care, the measurements found useful by the National Primary Care Collaborative[4] include:

- Number of days till third available *routine appointment* with each GP
- Number of days till third available *routine appointment* with Practice nurse
- % patients whose appointment was on their day of choice.

The selection of the third available appointment is to counteract the skew given to figures when one uses the first available appointment, which may only be there due to a last minute cancellation. This bears little relation to reality. As I have said earlier, we have expanded these measurements to most of the services offered to patients. This provided us with an intelligence that has proved very useful.

Many a time, I have followed a road atlas or the journey printout from my mapping software to prove the truth that *the map is not the terrain!* What appears so obviously on the map somehow bears no reality to the Welsh valley I am facing or the track I have

[4] The National Primary Care Development Team (part of the Modernisation Agency) http://www.npdt.org

just missed. Maps, at best, are only representation of reality – so are data. Data represent the reality of what we do and know as GPs and Practice Staff, it is not what we do or our knowledge. We must always be on our guard when interpreting practice data. When making the link from the numbers on the page to the eyes of our next patient, we must carefully consider the practice system in which we find ourselves.

We must not fall into the trap of predicting the future from the past; life seldom seems to go in a straight line.

> For a short time in the early seventies, the price of gold seemed to enjoy a constant increase in price. Being a recently qualified, but penniless, young doctor I listened night after night to the 'Money Programme' and the inexorable rise in the gold price, but had no money to enjoy the benefits.
>
> Then I thought of a plan: why didn't I buy a South African Krugerrand using my shiny new Barclaycard and sell it on before the end of the interest free period? I did some analysis on the situation, and looked at the past and current rise in the rate, and thought I could make, not a lot, but something with which I could put to buying another and so on ....
>
> Why hadn't others thought of this rather cunning plan, I wondered as I received my first glistening gold piece? It was so easy. Then I found out why! The price of gold tumbled much more quickly and suddenly than it had risen, and I was left with a considerable shortfall in my meagre saving!
>
> It is true the future can seldom be predicted from the past – and I won't tell you what happened to the rand!

It is much better to collect a little relevant information than spend masses of time collecting accurate information. When you know what is not working, use samples, not whole data sets. Be selective in collecting only that which you need to show you and your staff the direction of improvement; then make the same measurement in the same units to shown an improvement. The relevant information might not be quantifiable and numerate. It may be just as valuable if the qualitative information is gathered by asking the staff their opinion of the changes, or 'What is it like for you?'

But beware: collecting information and especially the information collected by others on your behalf, is not a value-free or a neutral process. It is all too easy for the person who is collecting the data to misunderstand the question of items being measured. This is not to say that we wittingly lie (though this has been known as well) but that as humans, if we feel a larger number of ticks on one side is more advantageous to us than more ticks on the other, there is a tendency for us to remember to count the former rather than the latter.

It is fundamental that the purpose of the data collection is understood by all involved to produce as standardised a collection as is possible. (Somehow communication seems to be a repeating theme!)

When writing about the data collection of change, a tool is the Plan Do Study Act Cycle, commonly abbreviated to the PDSA Cycle. It seems to me that this satisfies all that is necessary for safe, planned, sustainable change involving the whole Practice. PDSA Cycle methodology is dealt with in some detail later.

6   The people design principle

We have covered much of the detail around this principle already, but its importance justifies its development here.

In an organisation that is about to undergo change, the people who will be involved in these changes have the right to contribute to them. This is not only a matter of respecting, valuing and developing staff, but a very practical one too: your people are likely to hold the best idea! The changes necessary for the improvement you want for your Practice – whether they be in terms of patient access or the development of a new protocol for the treatment of hypertension – all are likely to be of a higher quality and carry a greater effect if they include the ideas of your staff.

People carry masses of information in their head; all they wait for is an opportunity to share that with you in suitable surroundings. The people who work in General Practice understand the problems of the Practice, and are more than likely to have valuable and constructive contributions for their solution. Staff do so much better when they own the solution.

Lastly, Practice staff are keen to get involved in data collection. They enjoy being responsible for projects and are usually fascinated by the results – especially when they see the relevance of their work in terms of a bigger plan.

7   Betterment time line

Put simply, this means that a solution to a problem should never be seen as a one-off. True, effective and sustained change is a planned, ongoing and continuous process. Change should have a timetable; individual changes should be seen in the context of each other; some may be simultaneous, but many are consecutive, building on the success, ideas and achievements that have gone before.

In exactly the same way as no protocol is complete without a review date, part of delivering a solution to a problem must include the intention of its re-examination at a fixed diary date. Even the best solutions became out of date; some stand the passage of time better than others, but all have *sell by dates*! It is important that the staff member – or GP, for that matter! – whose brain child the improvement was, should understand that the whole thing will be revisited at some time in the future with a view to further change and improvement.

As a doctor, I see evidence of the Law of Entropy every day, but still keep trying to fight it. I cannot understand how a desk I tidied last month becomes so cluttered *by itself* over the course of the month, undoing all my good work. Practice systems are like this, too.

> I remember speaking to a group of doctors, one of whom said that three years ago, he had operated an Advanced Access system. He had built up his Practice over the time – presumably attracting patients by his standards of access and care – but was finding that his original standards were no longer sustainable, and a backlog had developed.
>
> When asked if he had examined his system to identify the necessary tweaking it would undoubtedly need in that time, the answer was, "No."
>
> There must be few systems in medicine that do not need regular servicing and alteration over a period of three years. Societal changes themselves, let alone the increased appropriateness of treatment, would be enough to make further improvement an imperative.
>
> I smiled as I thought about the continuous painting of the Forth Railway Bridge! This is a constant job. By the time you have reached the end, the part you painted first is in need of repainting.

Why change does not work

No discussion about change would be complete without some consideration as to why change might fail. There are many examples of failure to make improvements which can deliver the necessary care to keep practice staff from leaving, doctors from dissolving partnerships and patient changing Practices. Let us consider and learn from a few of pitfalls we might face. These have been adapted from Kotter's work.[5]

No real mandate for change

Sometimes, the situation exists where although doctors and staff in a Practice give lip service to the need for change and improvement, no one is given the mandate to set the process in motion.

[5] *Harvard Business Review on Change: Leading Change: Why Transformation Efforts Fail*, 1991. John P. Kotter

One of the more influential partners feels he does not want to undertake yet another set of changes to the way he has worked for the last ten year. Perhaps he or she is contemplating retirement, perhaps he is nursing an illness or an ill member of the family, but for whatever reason, he simply does not want to change. This is known in the Practice, and no matter how hard the other partners try to lead the process, the staff know that the mandate of the influential partner has not been obtained and so the suggestions are not accepted.

This can be a difficult situation, and one that might have to be respected till the partner who is not lending his support to the change leaves the practice. Usually, however, some gain should be found in the solutions offered; if the processes can be seen to simplify and confer benefit to the individual, then they can often be persuaded to lend their support.

Not enough sense of urgency

Sometimes the problem is not so much getting the support of the leaders in a Practice, but is the fact that the urgency of the situation is not fully understood.

This urgency may originate externally in the form of some set of performance figures sent down from the Government or Primary Care Organisation, or from more clinically driven clinical audit measures in which a Practice might not be excelling. Certainly one of the best drivers is the sense of urgency that can develop when the actual standard of care delivered by a Practice is compared by the values held by that group; are they living to a standard of care of which they are proud?

Sometimes a Significant Clinical Event may be turned into a force for good, in that it creates a fear or concern that can only be dealt with by the introduction of Practice improvement that will make the error more difficult to repeat.

A Practice will find it easier to share these drivers when it is comfortable with itself, and can have frank and non-threatening conversation about Practice life as it really is – warts and all!

Guiding coalition is not strong enough

While I have no doubt the whole Practice should be involved with change, it is unreasonable to expect everybody in the Practice to have the same interest, commitment and strength of character to effect the changes. A Change Team, or Leadership Group, is required to be the engine for the exercise. The selection and composition of this group requires careful consideration.

Practices who are contemplating the idea of *working different-ly; smarter not harder* could do worse that prepare themselves by reading the work of Belbin[6] and the team roles he and his colleagues described. When forming the all important Practice Change Team, you will need at least one completer-finisher! One of the main functions of this group is to communicate, motivate and facilitate the Practice Team as a whole, so membership need not include everyone.

Having formed, however, this group must motor! It must have the individual and composite strength that is necessary to drive through the changes that come from the Practice as a whole.

It can be a lonely job, being a change agent, one that needs the sympathetic support of all the partners and senior staff. All of us fear change; most of us, on a personal basis, would very much rather continue to do that which we know we can do and do well, than experiment with new ideas, roles and practices. As well as providing support to the rest of the staff, the Change group needs to look after itself. Allowances must be made – perhaps in the form of periods of protected time or even away days.

[6] *Management Teams*, 2000, R. Meredith Belbin

Lack of vision

Change and its planned improvements often fail because of lack of vision. A vision may lack in terms of its clarity, content and communication.

A vision is not simply a plan to revamp the appointment system or to take on another partner; it is something about the overall plan of what the Practice will mean to its patients and staff in three years time. It is bigger than a series of projects; it is that of which doctors would be proud to look back on after their retirement; it is that which makes staff proud to say they work at their Practice.

This needs to be clearly articulated; it should be reduced to words on paper; it should be seen in the eyes of our staff; it involves the description of a culture.

But staff and doctors must believe that it is achievable, do-able and better than what exists at present. It needs to be owned by the whole Practice, not just the staff.

> Some years ago, the Mercheford House went through a low spell for which I accept my responsibility: the staff were not pulling together and the turnover seemed to have increased. Patients were still enjoying a high standard of care, but the surgery looked a little down at heel and unkempt. People seemed less pleased to be at work than they had been in the past.

It was felt that the starting point for change was to work on relationships within the staff, and the organisational culture in general. A series of monthly whole-staff meetings were set up where clinical and administrative matters were discussed. These were in advance of the now almost universal clinical governance afternoons.

Initially, the communication was mostly one way, but gradually the atmosphere changed. Staff members seemed to feel more empowered, and began to offer more suggestions and ideas.

When the time felt appropriate, a Workbook was prepared and each member of staff invited to complete one. The idea was to define the organisation and culture that they would wish for the Practice.

Out of this exercise came the Practice values as detailed in Chapter 2 and a Practice Plan for the following two years.

One point should be noted: for various reasons, none of the three partners completed a handbook! We had, however, absolutely no problems about accepting, signing up to and delivering the results – the vision had been communicated to the staff in the earlier meetings, and what had been reduced to paper was certainly something the doctors were delighted to share.

Like most other things in life, vision is not static; as change brings about a series of solutions to practice problems, the initial vision for the Practice begins to be realised. As this happens, the vision, which is essentially a future, idealised state, requires updating. The early vision took cognisance of the then current state of the Practice; as the Practice changes, so must the vision, for it must, by definition, arise from a different set of current Practice circumstances.

There must be a tension between the present state and the future vision. When this differential is small, the drive for change and achievement is weakened.

Under-communication

We all know the old adage about the three most important factors in successful change being:

1. Communication
2. Communication
3. Communication

Unfortunately for those of us who are poor communicators, this is actually true! True communication is what has happened when staff say, "Oh, *that's* what you mean! OK. Yes." When you have reached that point, people understand what it's all about; they are beginning to see the vision, the future, what their world might look like if the changes were to take effect.

It's a bit like learning to drive. When we first take to the road as a learner, we concentrate on what is directly a few feet in front of the car – the pavement or side-walk or the hole in the road. In due course, our gaze lifts, and we see the whole road opening before us and we anticipate possible scenarios. This is the effect of true and effective communication. We need to teach our staff to plan for the future.

Before a Practice can plan for the future, they must understand the final state vision – there must **be** a final state vision in the leaders' mind that can be communicated!

People must understand why they have been asked to collect specific data, where this will fit in with the grand plan. Not only will the value of the data be upgraded, but they are more than likely to be delighted to contribute to the realisation of the final vision.

In the final analysis, Practice staff want to know what is going on; they want to feel they are part of the grand design; they want to contribute to the improvement in the care of patients and be in tune with the values of the Practice; they want to become part of the success story of the Practice. This cannot happen unless they understand the plan; they will never understand the plan unless it is communicated to them.

True communication is a two-way process. Translated into other words, this might read: leaders must answer questions! Not all staff will see the point of collecting the numbers of telephone call that are taken each 15 minutes over the course of the day – unless they are informed of the end game plan and the part that their information will play in its achievement. But they will if it is explained to them!

The function of communication is to produce results – a good personal (or staff) relationship, a more efficient system, a happier practice…. The odd thing about good communication, however, is that after a few weeks, it is no longer a tool with which to increase the Practices audit marks, or a means to some other performance management end, but is enjoyed as an end in itself.

Without good communication, it is very difficult to achieve Advanced Access.

Not removing obstacles to new vision

Change produces anxiety, fear and resentment. Change often also requires the knocking down of walls, new space and the introduction of new equipment. This should be anticipated and planned for.

Some times, however, no matter what we say or do, change agents encounter apparently immovable objects that block all but minimal progress. These obstacles take different guises:

- **People**
  Poor or inadequate leadership, management, clinical staff, administrative staff
- **Things**
  Poor or inadequate premises, equipment
- **Finance**
  Poor or inadequate central resourcing, local resourcing
- **Organisation**
  Poor or inadequate Practice protocols, systems, procedures
- **Culture**
  Poor or inadequate Practice values, interpersonal relationships

Each of these areas is different and has different solutions. Some will involve Human Resource issues and professional guidance from those that are expert in that field; other problems may be corrected by training, or the use of temporary staff from other Practices; Practice culture can often be improved by whole Practice meetings or summer barbecues!

The point being made is that nothing should be seen as an immovable object.

A colleague who works in the secondary care sector confided a few locally used change strategies to me. These included:

- Meet every newly appointed consultant personally for introduction to the work of the change group
- Discuss their ideas for their speciality
- Provide resources/IT to make it happen
- This process may include any issue: office, secretary, equipment – just fix it to get their involvement!
- Invite new potential players to the change group, and introduce them to the team
- Demonstrate examples to support clinical practice
- Offer to publicise their arrival to GPs
- Arrange for them to meet GPs
- Marketing/private patients
- Identify the enthusiasts in any speciality
- Find means to supports change and the introduction of solutions to their problems
- Use the experience/credibility of clinicians (doctors, nurses, PAMs, etc.) to engage older consultants

This was a salutary lesson in terms of the Practice Introductory Pack and the induction of new staff members.

So far, we have skirted the issues of truly immovable objects but have concentrated on the prevention of such or the engaging of our resistant staff. Sometimes, however, people have to be side-lined; walls have to be build and money has to be spent. A return to the true values of the Practice makes this a little easier!

When contemplating this course, take appropriate advice before you start, perhaps from the HR department of a local Hospital Trust or the BMA.

Not planning for and creating short-term wins

In today's fast food society, folk like to see the benefits *now*! This is equally true in terms of Practice activity and change. When planning a change agenda for your Practice it is always a good idea to select an area that is known to be problematical and to fix it in the first few weeks or months of the project. Your staff – and that change-resistant senior partner or Practice manager – will hopefully see the benefit and become your firmest ally!

The only problem with quick fixes if that if they are based on *old think*, they can often make matters worse, or the backlog bigger!

We had agreed to perform a Practice audit of our elderly in terms of their last recorded blood pressure reading. It seemed a good idea at the time! But somehow, we never did get round to doing anything about it.

Time was passing, and the closing date was approaching. So, too, was flu vaccination time. Now there was a thought… Why could we not kill two birds with the one stone: why don't we check the BPs of all those coming for their flu vaccination – most of them belonged to the same target groups anyway.

On the face of it, this was a good idea. A nurse could do both if she had someone to help with the paperwork and recording in the patients records. It was done – an example of a quick fix, an early win!

What we did not foresee was the fact that the sight of a needle put so many patients' blood pressure up. Most of these fell again on follow-up. What was much worse, however, was the fact that the bolus of patients who needed their blood pressure checked at the BP Clinic created such a backlog, that it took our nurses months to catch up again!

This was a quick fix worked in an old system that had not the capacity to cope with the extra work. We did not make the same mistake the following year!

Early gains are only of value if they show the benefit in a change of system thinking; it is the new approach to work that we should be trying to demonstrate rather than the nose count of activity. Beware new wine in old bottles, and that sort of stuff.

Short-term wins must be planned for in the same sort of detail as the larger, more prestigious changes.

Declaring victory too soon

Sometimes, when the pain of change is dulled by the success of a major change, the imperative for further change disappears, and the organisation returns to its *status quo*. This is where a change time-line is so important. This is where the clear articulation of the final vision for the Practice is so fundamental. Change must not stop till the vision is realised in its entirety and this state will never be reached if the vision is regularly updated.

Not anchoring changes in the new culture

When a new form or procedure has been shown to be better than the old one, then remove and destroy the old forms and take away a central piece of apparatus used in the old procedure. Make it impossible to go back.

Many a valuable idea has failed because there has been an opportunity to return to what existed before. This means that the change agent's job is not over when the new procedure is in place; he or she must remain to ensure that it becomes firmly fixed in a new culture; he or she must work along side people who might want to slip back to their old ways, or not be quite as *au fait* with the new computer procedures as they made out at the meeting!

In conclusion

In conclusion, achieving Advanced Access probably should take a little longer than you think, though it does depend on your starting point. If you lead a Practice with a culture similar to that of a learning organisation, where staff and clinicians feel valued, are developed and are willing to contribute to change, you may be able to move quickly.

If, on the other hand, you have not started along that route, then the Practice culture is probably the place to start, and you have patients to develop the system from the ground up. (That is not to say that you may not be able to identify quick wins that might make a considerable difference early on, but in general, have patience.)

Such changes, as we have pointed out before, need all the involvement of all the practice staff. What is being described in this chapter is a way to produce the new way of providing medical care; doctors or Practice managers cannot do this on their own.

Equally, such a change cannot be brought about without realising the detail of your Practice's capacity and your patient's demand. Unless these can be seen to be balanced, then the old ways of systematised delays will prevail. It is only by understanding the precise nature of your patients' demands that they can be shaped and managed to coincide with the development and maximising of your Practice resources, the nature of which must be just as well understood.

Lastly, and something which leads us on to the next chapter, although each of us must select and develop the processes that suit our situations best, we must base them on a set of common principles that may be applied to any situation. We will go on to consider these.

Chapter 4

PDSA methodology

Introduction

Plan/Do/Study/Act is a form of audit cycle. The characteristics that make them a little different from typical audit cycles include the following:

- They are typically applied in circumstances where a large formal audit would not be possible or appropriate
- They frequently involve small numbers, e.g. perhaps only four or six patients
- They often involve individuals rather than the whole organisation
- They are seen, not as an end in themselves, but as a way to another piece of work

The magic PDSA cycle

ACT	PLAN
Changes to practice Communication of results Next cycle	Objective Questions/predictions What to do Data collection
STUDY	DO
Data analysis Comparison of data to predictions Lessons learned	Diary Unexpected observations Problems Initial results

Developing improvement

PDSA Improvement Cycles were reported by Donald Berwick,[1] referring to previous work. The idea is simple.

Someone has an idea that it is hoped might provide a solution to a particular problem or will start a process of change that will confer considerable gain to an organisation or an existing process. This idea is tested and refined by subsequent cycles.

As greater information, knowledge and understanding is gained, new procedures and system may be introduced, which in turn lead to sustained change.

One of the greatest benefits to encouraging the use of PDSA Cycles throughout an organisation is the change in culture that it can create. Staff at all levels are able to perform Cycles with respect to their own work, or can take part in the studies of others. This ensures that everybody's work is respected and seen as part of whole.

Not every PDSA Cycle will lead to an improvement; the outcomes of many have been buried, never to see the light of day! It is seldom, however that the work is totally wasted, for the

[1] A primer on leading the improvement of systems: *BMJ* 1996; **312**:619–622. Donald M. Berwick.

Langley GJ, Nolan KM, Nolan TW. *The Foundation of Improvement.* Silver Spring, MD: API Publishing, 1992.

Developing Practice improvement

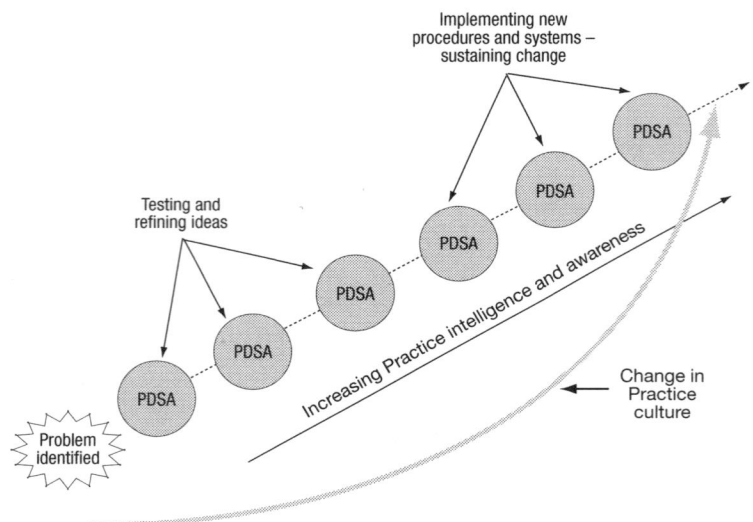

Developing Practice improvement

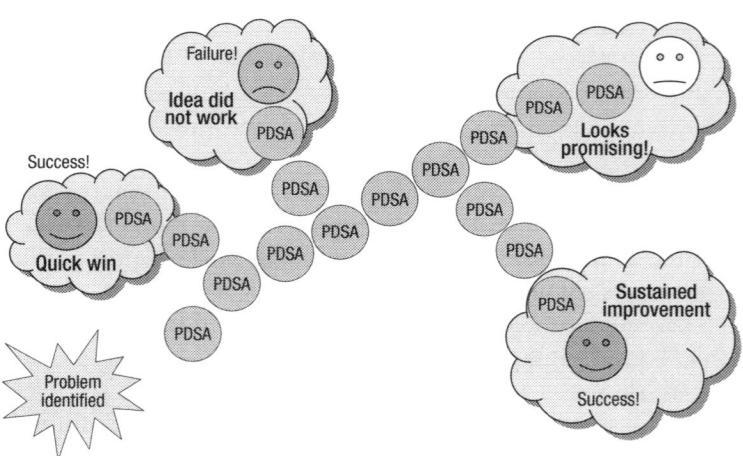

methodology can gather information that may be useful in other areas and can inform the work of other cycles.[2] It is the freedom that such short and frequent studies bring that make it exciting.

General rules

- Few PDSA Cycles should take longer than 3 or 4 weeks to complete.
- Most can be managed and reported using the four forms

[2] In fact, it can be argued that they are just as important as the successful cycles in that they can inform others of what failed to save them wasting time. On the other hand, it might inform another Practice of an idea that would work **for them!**

shown at the end of this chapter, with a couple of tables or graphs to demonstrate the results.

- Many PDSA Cycles should be in progress at the same time.
- Very few will require statistical analysis.

Description of process

As may be seen from the figure on page 73, there are four different parts to a PDSA Cycle: Plan, Do, Study, Act, and each of these will be considered in turn.

Plan

This refers to the thought that goes in to the exercise at its conception before anything is done, and seeks to answer the following questions:

1. Objective

What is that you are trying to do? If the work is wholly successful, what will the results help you to achieve? What ultimate changes in the way you currently do things are you working towards?

In many ways, this is a vision of a future situation, a final position, a *solution-after-next*. In all probability, it will **not** be addressed or achieved as a result of the planned study, which only focuses on a part of that fuller picture. Having a clear idea of your final aim, however, is vital to set your piece of work in the context of your bigger picture. It also helps communicate this end game to all the staff.

For example, if your ultimate aim is to reduce patients wait to see the treatment room nurse to less than 5 minutes, it is unlikely that your first PDSA Cycle will address all the issues needed to make this possible. You might run a series of different cycles looking at each of the many components involved in running an appointment system for the treatment room, one after the other. During this series of processes, it is important to keep your eye on the big objective so that your work has a context, rather than be side tracked to the many fascinating findings you will make.

- **Questions/predictions**

With respect to the piece of work you are planning, precisely what question are you attempting to answer? What are you predicting will happen as a result of this work?

This is the opportunity to be clear-cut and exact about the point of your study, and where it fits in with your overall **objective**. You should clarify your question, making it as precise as possible. In general, each PDSA Cycle should be used to answer a single question.

Being exact helps to ensure that the data you collect when you eventually perform the study is what you need in order to answer your original question.

It is also valuable to predict your results before you start collecting information. This not only helps you with the design of the cycle, but also heightens your understanding if the results are not those that you thought you would get. This in turn leads to a greater understanding of the problem you are addressing.

Another outcome is to test your current state of knowledge about your organisation. Often other areas of ignorance are highlighted which even at this point can lead to another set of Cycles.

3. **Plan to carry out the work (how, who, what, where, when)**
   This will mean being clear as to:

   • How precisely are you planning to do the work?
   • What methods will you use?
   • Who will be involved?
   • When will it start, and how long will the project run?
   • How will you share your results, and with whom?

It is most important to spend time, *walking* through your study in order to identify as many pitfalls as is possible before you start. By this I mean imagining yourself actually *doing* the study, *collecting* the information and even *analysing* it.

You will need to know who, if anyone, will be involved or participate in your study, and what they will do in terms of data collection. Have they agreed to participate? Do they understand what it is you are trying to do? You will need to explain the **question** you are setting out to answer, as well as the ultimate **objective** you have in mind.

You will have to be clear about exactly when it is to start, and how it will affect the organisation as a whole. You need to be clear as to how long you will need to run with the process. Some questions can be answered in a day or two, while some require a longer time scale, especially those that address less common situations.

It is important to understand that PDSA Cycles are not large, scientific trials, nor will the data be subjected to great statistical analysis. All that is needed is an answer to your original **question**. The study may have to be repeated some time in the future to ensure that any change made is successful, but it would be an error to make them long and complicated affairs from the start.

- **Plan for data collection:**
  Here it is about

  - How do you intend to collect data?
  - Exactly what information will you collect?

  You should have a clear notion in your mind as to how the study will be organised; how you will collect the information; the paper forms you will need to produce and how the data will be entered. You will need to be clear about what information is absolutely necessary to answer your original question or prediction. It is often tempting to collect as much information as possible, then to see what you can do with it at the end of the study. This can take your attention from the main aim of the study, and confuse the outcome.

  On the other hand, a study may be made ever so much more powerful by the inclusion of additional pieces of data. It is valuable to play with dummy data in the planning stages of a study, and even to go as far as to graph some random results in order to ensure that you are collecting the correct information that will enable you to answer the question you have posed.

- **Co-workers and integration:**
  At the bottom of the Planning page, there is a section to identify your co-workers. There is usually an information technology component to every PDSA cycle. People without knowledge of computers and the way they operate should seek to enlist the help of an IT literate colleague who can help them draw up their data collection forms, manage the data on a computer to make analysis and presentation of results easy. The name of these people should be recorded.

  In order to reduce the risk of duplication, that is different people doing the same work, all PDSA Cycles should have the approval of the co-ordinator. This is not a means of controlling who does what, but an attempt to ensure that the work done or currently in progress may be shared with others who are interested in similar areas, and to reduce duplication.

Do

The second area of a PDSA Cycle addressed the **DOing** of the project. This can be considered under four headings:

1. **Diary of project:** How did it go?

   In this section, notes should be made about the how the project went. Although day-by-day diary entries are usually unnecessary, it would be of value to others contemplating similar studies, to know the general details of how and what happened over the life of the project. This is also useful to you when designing future studies.

2. **Unexpected observations:** What did you find that you were not looking for?

   This section invites comments about the unexpected. Perhaps on the second day of the project you found that colleagues' attitude changed, either positively or negatively; perhaps you found that it was not possible to collect the data in the ways you had initially planned; perhaps simply calling attention to the problem led you and your colleagues to realise your overall objectives in another way.

3. **Problems:** What difficulties did you experience?

   The greater detail you can record in this section, the more information you will be able to use in future studies. Be as exact possible, listing the precise areas of difficulty. For example, when you or others look back at your work, if you have simply recorded the fact that you had 'computer problems', it may not be clear as to their exact nature. You may forget if they related to simply getting sufficient access to a PC, finding that you had difficulty with the program you were using to store your information or that your data was accidentally lost when the computer crashed!

4. **Results of the first look at the data:** What are your initial findings?

   In major scientific studies, it is often advisable that one should not take frequent 'peeks' at the data before they are properly collected. PDSA Cycles do not fall into this category of research. If the answer to your question is becoming obvious before the planned end of the cycle, then it may be sufficient for you to stop the **DOing** prematurely and move on to the **STUDY** part of the process.

On the other hand, the first few cycles may have been spurious and the benefits only noted later, as more data are collected. Caution always needs to be exerted when you make changes to your original plans.

Study

At the end of your cycle, all the data and information you have gathered needs to be analysed thoroughly. It is a mistake to take the information at face value, for there can often be discoveries other than the answer to your original question or prediction to be found in your body of collected data. Your **STUDY** of the results should be done systematically, perhaps with the help of a colleague.

1. **Data analysis:** What are your results and what do they indicate?
   Firstly, you should simply eyeball your results to gain a general impression:

   - Are they neatly recorded?
   - Have there been changes?
   - Where are the big numbers?
   - Where are the small numbers?

   Secondly, you should try to reduce your information to a graph. What does the graph of A against B look like? What relationship does C have to D? 'Every story tells a picture'; information is usually more easily understood when conveyed graphically. Again, you might want to involve a colleague to help in this.

   Thirdly, you should 'drill down' any area that looks different or interesting. If, for example, you notice a particular cluster of activity at an odd time of the day, you might want to look into this group, and review their particular circumstances – or to ensure that you have not made a transcription error!

   Lastly, you should go back over ALL the data you have gathered to make sure that you have not missed any interesting facts. This comes with experience, but there are few PDSA Cycles that will only throw up information that is restricted to your original question. Collected data often ask more questions than they were intended to answer.

2. **Comparison of data to predictions:** Did you get the results you expected?

Be honest! Do not alter your question or prediction in view of your results. Were your answers really those you predicted? If there were differences, why do you think they occurred? Did the methods you employed to collect the data best answer your question, or could you have done the study in a better way?

These types of questions are very valuable for future studies, and can save yourselves and others from wasting horrendous amounts of time making similar mistakes in the future.

3. **Summary of what you have learned:** What are your main conclusions?

This section is meant to contain the main conclusions from your study. There are usually only three or four such main points, though there may have been many interesting things found in the analysis of the data. The statements are those that you would use to summarise your conclusions when speaking to a disinterested colleague! They need to be short, pithy and to the point, but interesting enough to lead him or her to ask more of what you have been doing.

Act

The fourth and final part of a PDSA cycle is fundamental in as far as, if it is not completed, the exercise is likely to have been a waste of time.

1. **Changes to practice:** As a result of this study, what changes are you going to make to your practice?

The assumption made here is that you have been studying an area or work that holds some importance for you. The area will differ from person to person, and may not interest all (or even any) of your colleagues. It will, however, have interested you, which is why you set up the study in the first place.

This primary assumption means that you are faced with the need to make a decision with respect to the results you have obtained. In the face of the results, what changes do you need to make to the way you operate? What have the results highlighted that you should change in order to improve what you do? Which of the areas have been shown to be poor and need to be remedied? Put simply, what are you going to do about it?

It is important that you actually write these conclusions down, primarily for yourself in order to help fix the changes, but also for the benefit of anyone in your organisation that has been following the progress of your study – they will be able to anticipate what changes to their own pattern of work might result from what you intend to do.

2. **Next cycle:** What are you going to study next?
The last section of the worksheet has been included to help galvanise you to further action. It is highly likely that, having been interested enough to get this far, you will be asking more questions about how you work in the light of the conclusions you have reached. Jot them down! Bullet points will suffice, but if you have had an idea as to *how* your next cycle should be done, perhaps you should capture that as well before you forget it.

3. **Signing the work off:** Have you communicated your results with your colleagues?
The results of many studies are often not fully communicated. For example, it is important to inform your colleagues who helped you in the work. Not only will they value your thanks and acknowledgement, but they will be more likely to assist you in the future.

   Equally important is the possibility that your results might just give someone else the piece of information he or she needs to take their own work further, or lead to a new idea or question.

   Lastly, you should ensure that your piece of work is signed off by the PDSA co-ordinator.

Zones of challenge

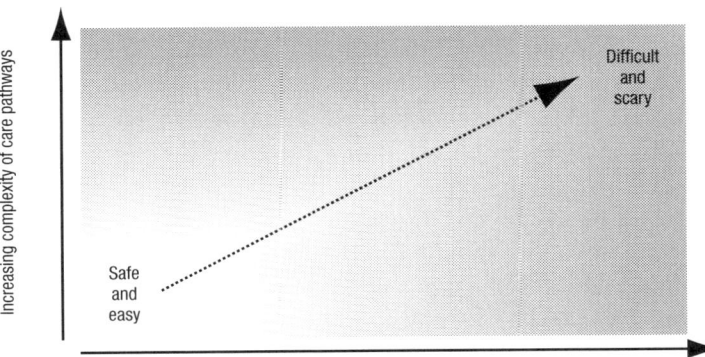

Note

While PDSA methodology is very powerful and has been associated with large scale and sustained change, there are areas where it can be more difficult than others. This does not mean that these methods should not be applied, but that the difficulties should be understood, predicted and anticipated, with solutions found ahead of the problems.

PDSA Cycles are easiest within single organisations when dealing with the improvement of simple processes. As both the complexity of the process under review increases, so does the difficulty in the organisation of the PDSA Cycle. This is simply to do with the size of the study and the number of components and people involved.

There is a similar increase in difficulty when the process being studied extends across different organisation, for example, Primary, Secondary and Social Care Organisations. The degree of Project Management and organisation increase exponentially. The methodology remains true, but the difficulty in its execution increases and more resolve and resources will be required.

Fortunately this will not often prove to be a problem within the confines of an individual Practice, but should be remembered when dealing with issues and pathways across a plurality of different Practices.

The PDSA form

The following four pages provide a suggested form format, though this may need alteration in the light of individual circumstances.

Name of Study:

PLAN for a PDSA Cycle for improvement

Objective:
- What are you trying to do in the long term?

Questions/predictions:
- What are you asking with this particular piece of work?
- What are you predicting will happen?

Plan to carry out the cycle: (who, what, where, when)
- How exactly are you planning to do the work?
- What Methods will you use?
- Who will be involved?
- When will you start, and how long will the project run?

Plan for data collection:
- How do you intend to collect data?
- Exactly what information will you collect?

IT person allocated to the study:

Work approved by: Date:

DO for a PDSA Cycle for improvement

Diary of project:
- How did it go?

Unexpected observations:
- What did you find that you were not looking for?

Problems:
- What difficulties did you experience?

Results of first look at data:
- What are your initial findings?

STUDY for a PDSA Cycle for improvement

Data analysis:
- What are your results and what do they indicate?

Comparison of data to predictions:
- Did you get the results you expected?

Summary of what you learned:
- What are your main conclusions?

ACT for a PDSA Cycle for improvement

Changes to Practice:
- As a result of this study, what changes are you going to make to your Practice?

Next Cycle:
- What are you going to study next?

Communication and thanks:
- Have you thanked everyone who took part in the study?
- Have you communicated your results to the Practice as a whole?
- Who else, perhaps in another organisation or Practice, might be interested in learning about what you have done?

Work signed off by: Date:

Chapter 5

Change principles

As with many other great things in life, Advanced Access is based on the application of a few, easily understood principles. In this chapter I should like to share these truths with you, and apply them to General Practice.

Mark Murray[1] speaks of high leverage changes and change concepts which can be applied to the redesign of medical care. I should like to present them in the specific context of delivering Advanced Access in General Practice

Basically theses ideas address the issues of practice intelligence – awareness and anticipation of what happens in our Practices.

> **Practice intelligence: awareness and anticipation**
>
> - Balance capacity and demand
> - Synchronise patient, provider, information and equipment
> - Predict and anticipate patient needs
> - Identify and manage constraints

Balance capacity and demand

This is really the bedrock on which successful and sustainable Advanced Access is based: it provides knowledge of what is expected of a Practice, and what the Practice has at its disposal to meet these expected demands. Unless this is based on facts that come from measurement, as opposed to impression, we end up being beaten by the shadows we fight.

Using PDSA methodology, the necessary information is fairly easily gathered. All aspects of demand should be mapped using simple tally counts against time. This must be extended, not simply to the demand for clinical staff but be seen to include measurement of the demands on individual receptionists, secretaries, administrative staff and management. Any demand that is not known about or understood cannot be shaped. All demand which has been understood can be, to a greater or lesser degree, shaped to conform to the resources available to meet it.

> **Understand the demand**
>
> - Predict daily/weekly/monthly demand
> - Understand the components of demand for services
>   - Numbers of follow-up appointments
>   - Numbers of same day appointment requests
>   - Patterns of phone calls: when and who deals with the calls
>   - Patterns of patients flow at reception
>   - Numbers of demand for Chronic Disease Management Clinic
> - Study the work content and flow of non-clinical staff

[1] Mark Murray, *Redesign the System* Learning Session Two – 31st October and 1st November 2001 http://www.doh.gov.uk/ero/accesscollaborative/learningsessions/lsessiontwo/ls2.htm

Know your resources

- Map out the times and hours worked by all staff
- Keep a record of skills and knowledge that staff have but that are not used in the Practice
- Learn the aspirations of all your staff
- Check the timetabling of all rooms, and list times – and duration – of all Clinics
- Ensure that a current inventory and the location of equipment is known to all staff

Synchronise patient, provider, information and equipment

- First a.m. and p.m. appointments to start on time
- All necessary information and paperwork for decision present at time of decision
  - At time of consultation
  - Checking investigation results
  - Practice meetings
- Regular equipment and stationery checks

In the same way, we require to know what resources and tools are available to meet these demands. As we are all aware, staff are our greatest – and most expensive – resource. Often, many of them are not working to their optimal potential; many have had previous training and skills of which the Practice is unaware, but which may be all that is necessary for a successful change solution to be implemented. A good staff appraisal system would go a long way to ensuring that such a waste of talent or expertise does not occur.

Synchronise patient, provider, information and equipment

This principle is one of the strongest and most effective at creating clinical space and time within a Practice – and it is common sense as well!

Before GPs can complain that they are overworked, they must be sure that they start on time! This is probably the biggest reason why doctors get home late, why so many patients unnecessarily crowd our waiting rooms and why reception staff feel so pressurised.

How can we as doctors insist that all other clinical and administrative staff arrive on time while we start when we wish?

Basically, everything I need as a nurse, doctor, receptionist, secretary should be to hand when I deal with the patient who is likely to require them. There should be no unnecessary down time.

I am by no means brave when it comes to visiting dentists; but when it comes to oral surgery, that's even worse! I was once advised to have an apicectomy – a dental root clearance from the inside.

Bravely, I went to the oral surgery unit where the procedure was explained to me; I had a surface anaesthetic – and my dread by this time was clear to all as I lay down on an operating table with my head in what seemed like a rubber vice, with my face hidden from view.

The surgeon proceeded to infiltrate the local anaesthetic then made the incision – well at least that was not painful, I thought; my peri-dental tissues were cleared with something no respectful GP would ever have in his surgery; the surgeon asked for the reamer (?) only to find that the bit was not to his liking; it was not the one he wanted; he had wanted the 3mm variety which allowed a more acute angle at the neck!

Twenty-five minutes later he re-started the operation. What might have been a 15-minute procedure lasted nearly 45 minutes. I noted that there were a greater number of patients in the waiting room when I left than when I arrived! I doubt if the poor surgeon would catch up on that half hour for the rest of his day, and most of his patients would incur another 25 minutes in the waiting room.

The point of this story is not to make complaint against my oral surgeon colleague – there is often much more behind a delay in medicine than meets the eye; but to illustrate the fact that precious clinical time can be wasted if we do not have everything that is necessary to hand when we need it.

This is by no means a secondary care phenomenon; it would not be the first time a GP has kept a patient waiting on a treatment room couch for a rectal examination, only to be offered an apology that there were no sigmoidoscopes available. As well as being poor medicine, this is a complete waste of clinical time.

The same is true for the more obvious situations where patients keep appointments with their GPs who do not have the necessary hospital reports or investigation results.

It is when receptionists can save a minute here and a couple of minutes there that they can be employed to do some more clinical type of work; it is by being efficient that nurses can pull work from doctors; it is by having everything to hand that doctors can save time during their surgeries to be able to see patients on the day they wish to be seen. All of this saved time, from all parts of the organisation can then be translated into clinical time.

Predict and anticipate patient needs

Having increased our intelligence of Practice activities, we must communicate this information to all concerned. Different pieces of information should be shared in different ways and with different frequencies. Standing items on the agendas of these meeting should reflect the timely importance of this data.

Levels of communication

In all but the smallest Practices, meetings are a necessary part of medical life. Their frequency, composition and content will vary, but they must be seen by the staff to be structured, disciplined, important and worthwhile.

The following are a few thoughts on possible scenarios.

Predict and anticipate patient need

- Levels of communication
  - Monthly meetings
  - Weekly meetings
  - Huddles
  - Communication shortcuts
- Plan for the predictable
  - Common things happen commonly
- Plan for the unexpected
  - Emergency medical and stationery supplies
  - Fax, phone numbers, delegation to staff

- **Monthly meetings**

  Items concerned with planning activity over the next few months should be covered regularly as monthly meetings. There are very few Practice matters that cannot be shared at whole staff meetings. Monthly data relating to the previous months should be discussed to enable all staff to understand the larger picture

  Minutes of these meetings should be kept and made available to staff, either in paper form or on the Practice intranet site if one exists.

- **Weekly meetings**

  The agenda for weekly Practice meetings has more to do with the day to day running of the Practice, and may simply involve senior management. It is good policy, however, to put out some form of notes or bulletin afterwards to keep folks up to date. Any staff sensitive and personal information may be kept for the minutes, which should not be routinely shared, but reflect the whole content, context and detail of the meeting.

  This detail is important for clinical governance purposes and should be as exact as possible. It should be checked in draft form as well as at the subsequent Practice meeting.

- **Huddles or corridor meetings**

  Huddles refer to the small, often spontaneous and unstructured, meetings that take place throughout the day when staff have information to pass on that improves the running of the Practice.

  It may be something to do with the level of patient demand that day, the fact that the Practice is running low in tetanus vaccine or that the local hospital is on red alert. The knowledge of such almost trivial pieces of information enables the Practice to run smoothly and efficiently with few stoppages. This all helps to create the environment where patients can see the doctor of their choice on the day of their choice.

- **Communication shortcuts**

  There are all sorts of examples of communication shortcuts, often involved non-verbal communication. All have the common result of helping to keep the team up to date with what is happening in the Practice on a moment by moment basis, as well as encouraging a team spirit that enables it to function better when things go wrong.

  An electronic bulletin board can be a useful idea as long as it is kept up to date. These may be identified on a Stop Press facility, where snippets of day to day information are posted.

A more formalised site like a Practice Newsletter, which is updated on a monthly basis, is equally useful.

Plan for the predictable

It is amazing that in many Practices, doctors find themselves searching around for request forms, MSU bottles and the like. They and their staff should know that these will be needed, and simple systems should be in place to make sure that everything is to hand in order to save time which can be spent on clinical care. Responsibility for this can be delegated down the practice organisation.

Planning for holidays in terms of medical and administrative cover; succession planning for staff and doctors approaching retirement: all of these are predictable and should come as no surprise. The heavy work load after a Bank Holiday or annual leave can be anticipated and should be planned for.

Plan for the unexpected

The same is true for the things that happen infrequently, but are of a more unexpected nature. An example might be patients presenting with severe asthma. These are often met with a sudden searching around for a nebuliser and Salbutamol nebules. The time to check the expiry date of emergency medical supplies is not during the emergency! If supermarkets can organise the regular checking of sell by dates, then so can General Practice.

The increasing use of a shared telephone book on a Practice intranet make it easy to share the same set of telephone numbers. All staff should be trained to phone ambulances, etc., again to save time that may be given to patients.

Identify and manage constraints

When planning for change, one or the basic principles we should all adopt is to ensure that everyone is working to the highest level they can in relation to their knowledge, training and professional qualifications. As I have pointed our before, this can never be a fixed stat of affairs as we are all capable of learning and doing more. It is fairly easy to identify a constraint – there is usually dissatisfaction, a queue, a pile or a delay before it!

Identify and manage people constraints

- Person constraint
  - All work to highest level of skill, expertise and professional qualifications
  - Only do that which adds value to patient care
    - ○ Carers should only do that which only they need to do
    - ○ Training and staff development keeps this from being a static situation
  - Temporary shifts in work between professionals
    - ○ Doctor, nurses, prescription clerks, secretaries, Practice managers, etc.

People constraints

Practices who invest in training and development for their staff are more likely to deliver Advanced Access for they will usually have a skill-mix that is suited to the work they have to face.

Many former medical and nursing tasks may be delegated to nurses and care assistants respectively as long as the following are respected:

1. The staff member is specifically trained to perform the task.
2. The staff member is happy that he or she is competent to undertake the task.
3. There is a direct line of responsibility for the staff member and his/her work.
4. There is adequate support at hand if ever required by the staff member.

As a general rule, staff members – including medical staff – should only do that which only they can do: everything that can be done by others, and which does not need a particular level of qualification should be delegated down, according to the principles set out above.

Another way to think on this is that everyone in a Practice setting should add value to patient care when they are in contact with patients in a way that, as a result of their qualifications and training, only he or she can.

Some of these shifts of workload can become permanent, but often the system requires only temporary assistance. This takes us back to the picture of the bale of hay – once your name is on it, it is your responsibility. The Practice may have to wait for the work to be done, but it can only be done by the chap whose name is associated with the work.

Normally, my secretary types the notes I dictate about patients I see in surgery. Occasionally, when she is becoming pressurised with unplanned work coming from other directions, she will ask me if I would enter my own notes onto the computer to reduce her work temporarily till she catches up again or till her secretarial colleague returns from vacation. Not a problem. Work flows from her to me for a few days. She will let me know when she is able to take the work back.

This freedom to allow the loose hay from the haystack to be worked on by the most appropriate member of staff is a very powerful tool in the creation of clinical time in which to allow the delivery of Advanced Access.

Process constraints

The constraint in most Practice systems is usually the doctor. It is important therefore that he should only do that for which his skills and qualifications are needed. The nature of work going into his room should be that that only he can do.

When faced with this situation, any inspection of the suitability of the work for the GP should be placed before it arrives at his room. In other words, it is a waste of the doctor's time deciding if the work is his or not; this inspection step should have come earlier in the process, thereby allowing the GP to do what it requires a GP to do.

With this in mind, and respecting the need for privacy and confidentiality at the reception desk, the work flowing into General Practice should be diverted as soon as possible, and certainly before it comes to the clinical staff.

Admitting that the majority of the work in General Practice is self-generated by the clinicians themselves, the best and most effective method of dividing the flow is at the time of the original consultation or Chronic Disease Management Clinic visit. This is where changes of practice, for example, the shifting of follow-up appointments for patients with hypertension or asthma from the doctor to the nurse is best made, rather than waiting to decide when the patient is presenting for the follow-up appointment, not knowing the clinic at which to book.

> **Identify and manage process constraints**
>
> - Process constraint
>   - Separate types of flow
>   - Patient
>   - Contacts
>   - Personal
>   - Phone
>   - Treatment room
>   - Care assistant
>   - Chronic Disease Management Clinics
>   - GPs
>   - Phone
>   - Investigations
>   - Repeat prescriptions
>   - Medical advice and information

Change concepts

In an effort to create capacity or clinical space, consider the following principles. Remember that the concept should be a common haystack of work faced by the Practice, not individual bales of work with the names of individuals attached to them. These principles should be applied across the Practice so as to save time and work anywhere in the system in order to translate it into clinical space.

Eliminate waste

- **Eliminate things that are not used or needed**
  I would judge that in every Medical Practice, staff – including doctors – collect information or faithfully follow instructions that have lost their relevance and value years ago. Habits that were important to staff when they first started and became

almost a status symbol are being continued for absolutely no reason. The time spent in these activities could be used much more productively.

> Years before we were computerised, I had instituted a daily count of the patients I had seen. At the beginning, the data were interesting, and showed the general activity of the Practice, but when we became computerised, no one thought to inform the staff member. This only stopped when I took away the battered old notebook containing the figures that were no longer used.

We must always look to ensure that each member of the Practice spends their time in sensible and productive ways, ensuring that everything brings value to our patients.

- **Stop multiple entry**
  Consider having shared, centralised files which may be accessed by all the Practice. For example, a single Practice telephone directory, or list of local consultants stored in an intranet site could save the receptionists from being interrupted by doctor who have forgotten the number of ambulance control.

  Multiple entry of information is a much greater problem in the secondary sector, but our Practices should be scoured regularly to ensure that this waste of time has not crept in.

- **Eliminate overkill**
  Although there are situations where great detail is valuable, especially in note taking and note keeping, sometimes we can be guilty of overkill that makes getting to the important facts difficult. We should only do that which is clinically useful, necessary and can be used in clinical decision-making. Overkill is a waste of resource.

  Perhaps the area where doctors can be most guilty of overkill is that of screening. In an effort to ensure that every elderly person receives what he or she needs, we ask all our elderly all the questions on a questionnaire. Not only are many of the questions irrelevant, but patients can feel quite insulted.

  Care should be segmented so that everybody gets only what he or she needs; patients should only be asked relevant questions. The use of trigger questions can help in this process, something which elevates the importance of questionnaire design.

- **Sample**
  From what has been said about PDSA Cycles, the value of sampling should be clear. It allows the greater understanding

about so many more areas in Practice – a little about a lot is usually much more useful than a lot about a little.

Successful PDSA Cycles have been based on as few as 5 to 10 patients; that may be all that is required to confirm, refute or develop a hunch.

- **Remove intermediaries**
  There are two ways of removing intermediaries:

  a) Give the task to the correct person in the first place; or
  b) Enable the person facing the task to complete it in its entirety.

  Examples of both of these principles have already been described, but perhaps one that has not been emphasised is the value of doctors speaking to patients directly using the phone, rather than relaying messages through secretaries. Shared computers make the sharing of the necessary information a lot easier.

- **Delegate fearlessly but properly**
  Delegation involves communication and sharing of intention before work is delegated; it needs training to ensure the person involved has the necessary knowledge and skills and agreement that by both trainee and trainer that this point has been reached; it requires a monitoring system to be in place with quality checks; and it involves having a clear and direct line of responsibility to a more senior worker in times of difficulty and uncertainty. If these principles are in place, there is almost no limit to the value of delegation.

  Some people, both clinical and administrative, find it more difficult to delegate than others. This is for different reasons, which include the following:

  - Fear of upsetting the patient or colleague
  - Lack of confidence in the one to whom the work is being given
  - Lack of confidence on the part of the one who is responsible for the work shift
  - Fear of loss of control over the process as a whole
  - Fear of being de-skilled
  - Unhappiness about loosing part of the job that they like doing.

  Coaching skills have a lot to teach us with respect to the area of delegation. There are several excellent short texts that explain the principles and are well worth reading.

Improve workflow

- **Synchronise care and actions**

  Start on time; ensure that everything that is needed is to hand. Requesting a copy of a direct breast referral from your secretary involves your time as a doctor and her time bringing one through to your room. If you arranged a small stock pile in your room, she could get on with more productive work, and you could save time to see other patients.

- **Minimise hand-offs**

  All staff should be trained to deal with all of the common issues presented to them, for example making an appointment, organising patient transport or running off a repeat prescription. This is not to argue that one should not have 'specialists' in the Practice, but it can save a lot of time, especially on Saturday mornings if all staff can perform the more frequently needed tasks.

- **Move steps closer together**

  An example of this might be referral letters and when to write them. It seems that a common habit for doctors is to 'batch' activities such as this to a 'more suitable time'. This usually results in a delayed referral and a content that not does always bear a complete resemblance to what was in the mind of the referring doctor at the time the patient was seen.

  By much the better plan is to either dictate the letters immediately after the patient is seen, or allow sufficient time at the end of surgery to clear off all correspondence. The increased efficiency and improved patient care comes from moving the steps closer together, allowing time for the process as required.

- **Remove bottlenecks**

  Bottlenecks need to be identified first. Like constraints, they are usually quite easy in that they are always preceded by delay – queues of patients, piles of notes, stacks of correspondence...

- **Automate**

  The value of automation has increased with the increased use of computers. Mail merge and computerisation of repeat prescription systems can save a great deal of work around group correspondence.

  On the other hand, having a sheet of pre-printed address labels can save a lot of time as well! Manual automation still has its place in Practice.

- **Do tasks in parallel**

  Often it takes as much time to do two tasks as one. When the second task belongs to another department or carer, his or her time can be saved, the overall resources of the Practice increased, and this will eventually translate in clinical time.

- **Use *pull systems***

  A *pull system* draws work from the future to the present; whereas a *push system* pushes work from the present to the future.

  A doctor who uses *pull* principles will say things like, "If I've got to do it anyway, I might as well do it now; it will save me time in the long run" or, "I'll do it now, as nurse will need to do it next week, and that will mean another trip for you" – and another appointment, work for the receptionist to make the appointment and to check the patient in and an appointment with nurse that might be given to another patient!

  A doctor who uses the *push* principle will tend to put work off till a later date; he will have a pile of letters to write, as he says he likes 'batching his work' and will frequently say to patients, "I think you should make another appointment and I'll see to that then."

  Pull systems helps to ensure space, time and resource for the future. It increases the ability to deal with problems as they crop up without having to work harder, or squeeze patients in. It develops a feeling of being in control.

Optimise the work environment

- **Access to information**

  - Training
  - Cross-training

  These concepts extend the cultural values of investing in and developing Practice staff. It also creates an increased efficiency that reduces bottlenecks and handoffs, where work is put in bundles for someone else to do.

  > We have a reception clerk who spends the vast majority of her time managing the Practice's repeat prescription system. This has meant that her detailed knowledge has reduced the number of errors in our prescribing, decreased the delay in processing repeat prescriptions and allowed us to introduce clinical checks before items are issued.
  >
  > But we also have another colleague who can step in to take her place during holiday and sickness.

- **Manage variation**
  - Standardise
  - Contingency plans
  - Manage peak demand

This is a problem for doctors! Getting doctors to agree to do the same thing is only half as difficult as getting them to do the same thing! It is possible, never the less, to get doctors to reduce the variation in the way they do things. Protocols help this. It should be noted that the essence of democracy and agreement everyone has to get something he or she wants from a protocol, while at the same time agreeing to concede in other areas. This can be a time consuming process, but it pays dividends in the long run by saving time.

Accident and disaster hit the best run Practices. Flu epidemics can create large increases in demand, while enforced absences can cause sudden and unexpected reduction in capacity. Both should be planned for at Practice meetings.

Individual, day to day planning is also of value and should help to avoid: "Doctor, when should I book patients when your appointments have all been taken?"

Standing instructions to receptionists that patients should be automatically warned if the doctor is working more that 20 minutes late is not simply good manners, but helps to reduce the paperwork involved in dealing with patient complaints, and may well result in some patients re-scheduling their appointments.

Conclusion

When written down in simple form, these change principles may seem facile and obvious, but it is amazing how many of us violate them in the way we deliver care. Ignoring them, results in a considerable waste in resources. This in turn results in an imbalance of resource and demand that makes us ask for more money for new staff. Unless we can change the system, it is unlikely that increased money, staff or other resources will make any but a short-term improvement.

Chapter 6

Frequently asked questions

Do you give specific appointment with individual times to all your patients?
All patients are given appointments – except during the *fire-breaks*.

In the evening, one of our local pharmacies remains open till 6.30 p.m. In order to ensure that patients can collect their prescriptions before closing time, we invite them to attend at 5.30 p.m. to ensure minimal delay

Do each of the partners have the same appointment template?
No. Two work to an 8 patients/hour schedule while the other is more comfortable with a rate of 6 patients/hour. What is important is that each health care professional works as near as is possible to his or her own periodicity.

You seem to imply that you receptionists are able to update you as to the daily pressures for appointments. Do you mean that you and your Receptionists form a team?
Our Receptionists know to contact the GP directly when they realise demand is increasing. Our Practice managers are involved when it comes to changing the formal appointment templates, but any minor response to day to day demand is usually settled between the receptionist and the GP.

Information about the number of visits is also put on the screen, as are details of any meeting the GPs might be attending. This helps to keep everyone abreast with what is happening in the Practice on a daily basis.

There must be days when you want to reduce your work to allow you to go to meetings, etc. Do you have this flexibility?
The answer is, yes to both questions. Advanced Access has two guiding principles:

* The receptionists should not allow an undue build up of prebooking, which constitutes backlog; and,

- Patients should see the doctor of their choice on the day of their choice.

Although it is difficult to make the distinction in words, two concepts must be kept separate. The first is the cardinal proof of Advanced Access, that is actually seeing the doctor of choice on the day of choice, irrespective when the appointment was actually allocated to the patient. The second are the issues around when that appointment was allocated, i.e. on the day of the request, or on another occasion.

In Mercheford House every patient who phones before 4.00 p.m. requesting an appointment on the day of the phone call will be seen on the day of that request. If the request is for an appointment on a day in the future, or one which is seen to be already heavily booked, the patient will be given the option to phone back on the particular day – when they will be given an appointment as per the above rule – or be offered one on an alternative day.

In practical terms, what this means is that on the days after a doctor has been on call overnight, has a Primary Care Organisation meeting or needs to keep a dental appointment, he can block off his appointments as 'book on day'. This flags to the receptionist that patients who want to be seen on the day must wait till that day to phone up for an appointment. This goes a long way to protecting the demand on a particular day; those patients who want the prior certainty of knowing that they definitely have an appointment, they might prefer to book on another day.

Some doctors have a standard rule that patients may pre-book up to 30% of the daily available appointments; after this patients requesting to be seen on that day will always be seen on that day, but they will need to wait till the day before they can confirm their appointment. The introduction of this apparent uncertainty often makes patients select another day on which to see their doctor.

The principle of planning and intelligence is paramount; receptionists must be kept up-to-date with what the GP and nurses are planning; they must function as a team.

But you must have had surgeries that have over-run?
Yes, I suppose I must; but they are certainly less frequent that they used to be. I judge my day by the 1.00 p.m. and 7.00 p.m. television news programmes. If I get home to hear these programmes, I know I am working to time! I might choose to do my visits

before lunch, but this is a matter of choice. Most days, other than when my partners are on holiday, I can manage to hear most of the news programmes.

My personal strategies are to use the fire-breaks I have already described, or on really bad days, to fit in patients between the normally booked appointments as *extras*. This is the exception rather than the rule.

The important point I should like to make is that my frequency of 'bad' days are much lower than they used to be. I have not been regularly over-run.

I have been taught that a consultation should last for at least ten minutes. How can you deal with all your patient's problems in 7½ minutes?

I cannot, and I do not. What I said was that, on average, I saw eight patients an hour. This means that some only need 3 or 4 minutes, while some take 14 or 15 minutes. On average, I can comfortably see 8 patients an hour. If someone obviously needs a greater amount of time spent with them, I arrange for them to attend at the end of surgery, and simply run over.

Each of us has our own, natural periodicity at which we see patients. We should respect this rather than some externally or arbitrarily applied timetable.

What happens when you come back after your holidays?

In Mercheford House, the week after a doctor's holiday is kept totally free of appointments – except perhaps the first four on a Monday morning. Patients are then free to phone up on the day of their choice to see the doctor of their choice; the doctor and staff know that there will be enough space as the appointment schedule is free.

Did all the doctors move to Advanced Access at the same time?

No. When I attended the First Workshop for the 2nd Wave of the National Primary Care Collaborative, I did some calculations that seemed to show:

- I was providing slightly in excess of the number of appointments my lists size needed. This was based on the fact that 0.7 to 0.8% of a registered practice population tried to contact their doctor on any single day.
- I regularly had excess capacity at some time during the week, usually on a Thursday, which indicated that by developing nurse-led clinics and the transfer of patients from my surgery

to nurses had already worked, and I was balancing my capacity and demand on a weekly basis. All I had to do was to shift and balance them on a daily basis.

On the Monday morning following the 1st National Primary Care Collaborative, I arrived in surgery before my Practice manager who had been at the collaborative meeting as well, and intimated to the staff that I would see patients on the day they wished to be seen. As you can imagine, I had the usual incredulous remarks. "You want what? You'll be snowed under! Where do you want to put the extras?" etc. Fortunately it worked, and my hunches were correct; I did not have a huge backlog, and the weekly numbers, although a little greater for the first two Mondays, settled, and I have never looked back.

As far as partners were concerned, one was due to retire in the following April. He never did get round to Advanced Access – but his replacement, on the other hand, thought it a good idea and has worked in similar ways to mine since he joined the Practice!

My third partner was a little more diffident. He felt happy with the way he ran his appointments and did not want to change. Unfortunately he sustained an accident, and was away from work for a few months. We were not able to get as much locum cover as we wanted, but because the remaining two of us did not have a backlog ourselves, we were able, with a little locum help, to keep pace with the increased work, and began to work off his remaining backlog. On his return, he was able to start with only a few booked patients, i.e. the same backlog as the rest of us.

There are minor differences in the way we operate, in that two of us prefer to clear the bulk of the appointments in the first half of the day in order to ensure getting away on time; while the other is happier to spread the work a little more evenly with the threat of working a little longer in the evening. Basically, however, the systems are the same, and patients would be hard pressed to spot any differences.

I can understand that the Advanced Access could work in single-handed Practices, or where doctors have their own lists of patients. What about Practices that operate a shared list system?
This is a fascinating point. While at one of the NPC collaborative meetings, I met a GP who had started to deliver Advanced Access before I had. He ran a shared lists system, and used to get asked exactly the opposite question: "It's OK for you; you have a shared list. What about those of us with single lists?"

During conversation with him, both of us answered in the same vein. We considered it easier to deliver Advanced Access in the system with which we were familiar, but that the other's system might have made it more difficult!

I think it boils down to horses for courses. We all know the product we want to deliver – Advanced Access, enabling patients to see the doctor of their choice on the day of their choice; we all know the principles on which such an achievement will be based. These things are shared. The difference is the processes we adopt to get there. These will be unique to each Practice. I can describe the product and the principles, but only you in your own Practices can work out the processes you will use – though some of them may look similar to the experiences I have described as being used in Mercheford House.

What about the popular or unpopular doctor? Giving patients a free choice would overwork some partners, and leave others with time on their hands? How do you get round that one?
This can be a delicate matter. The answer is certainly not to concentrate on personality, but on the principles of demand and capacity.

a) In the first instance, it might be useful to run a PDSA Cycle to look at the types of problems presented to individual GPs. This may show that some doctors attract more than their fair share of problems that might be transferred to nurse-led Chronic Disease Management Clinics.

b) A second Cycle might be used to look at any variation in recall patterns, demonstrating that some doctor ask more patients to come back than others in absolute terms; or the difference might be the shorter intervals of return. Standardisation across all partners might help this.

c) Some doctors find it more difficult to ask patients to leave them to see either nurses or other doctors than others. PDSA Cycles are able to identify a form of words which works and which are acceptable to both doctor and patient.

d) The promptness which a doctor regularly starts his morning and afternoon surgeries often plays an important part in the apparent popularity stakes, as does setting a realistic length of time for the duration of his consultations.

e) Occasionally, training needs require attention, as does the use of other colleagues; some doctors finding it more difficult to delegate than others.

f) Sometimes it is the way we organised our day that makes things less efficient. Good secretarial help can go a long way to improve this.

g) Sympathy should be shown to GPs whose personal professional habits appear to cause more work than their colleagues. In the last analysis, however, it is the patient, not the doctor, whose needs should be served; this may not always allow us as individuals to spend the time we want on certain clinical situations.

h) The development of Practice protocols can help to influence those whose behaviour is not in line with Practice policy.

We have a nurse who will not change. What do you do then?
I believe that having good nursing staff is the mainstay of Advanced Access; a capable, knowledgeable and trustworthy nursing colleague is worth her weight in gold. When one is faced with a member of staff who has contributed well to the care of patients in the past, but who, for whatever reason, is not up to the current clinical demand, sympathy rather than retribution is the order of the day. Often the person concerned knows of her problems, issues that have caused her anxiety for some time.

My first advice is to talk! Try to identify the real issues. They may include training, knowledge, confidence, illness, fear of illness, having not recovered from a past incident, or the way it was handled. Understanding often paves the way to change and success.

In the truly rare circumstances where there is a straightforward lack of cooperation and refusal to 'play', the advice of a local Human Resources Department should be sought before becoming embroiled in confrontation and employment law.

We have a senior partner who will not allow change. We have talked about these things, but he simply says he is too old to change, and gets very defensive. We have tried, but he will not even let us develop a BP Clinic.
Difficult. As far as the Partnership is concerned, he has similar rights as the other partners, but as far as patient care is concerned, he has the responsibility to deliver as high quality and efficient services as possible.

My first thoughts would be to approach the situation as I described for the nurse. Explanation and two-way communication can often help to resolve matters. Showing him or her that he will not be involved in more work and that all he needs to do is to enjoy the benefits of the changes often helps.

Sometime, it must be admitted that some Partners are able to block change permanently; the only answer in these circumstances may be to wait for the doctor to retire!

What about money? You have not mentioned the fact that all these changes will mean new staff, new resources. Where is the money going to come from? The Primary Care Organisations?
I'd like to answer to that in two different ways:

a) I have worked with change programmes in Primary and Secondary Care for some time now, and I have never come across an important change that was blocked for the want of money. I have seen many that did not even attract pump priming. Change happens because people want it to happen. I have seen money come in as a reward for change in order to develop other improvements, but that is a separate matter.

b) The second point I would like to make is that when making a case for increased Practice resources, whether they be medical, nursing or other staff, we must be pretty clear that our current staff are being used to their maximal and optimal limits. Before we ask for more, let's empty our buckets of all the unnecessary work they may contain; do this for all practice staff; and then look again at who does what. It will be truly amazing what a unified, planned approach will deliver.

It is true that in some circumstances, there is an absolute shortage of space, personnel or kit; in these circumstances, where demand is truly greater than supply, a balance can never be attained. There must be few circumstances, however, where capacity cannot be increased by applying the principles we have described.

I have heard that some Practices provide same day booking. Is this the same as Advanced Access?
Yes and No in my opinion.

If patients are getting to see a doctor on the day they choose, then I suppose this is Advanced Access. I know some Practices that only allow patients book up morning appointment in the morning, and have to wait to the afternoon before they release their afternoon appointments. Others only allow booking up to 24 hours later – in other words, a patient may phone or present in the morning for an appointment that morning or afternoon or the morning of the next day, but no later.

Some Practices have found this to be a problem, and have noted that their complaints have actually increased. Previously, the complaint was about waiting for 1, 3 or 21 days to see their GP; now it is that they cannot make an appointment for 3 days hence, but have to accept the uncertainty of waiting till the morning arrives, running the gauntlet of the phones and potentially having to set the whole day aside to see their doctor. At least when they had to wait, they knew the time at which they were going to be seen and could plan their day accordingly.

There is a balance to be struck between what is manageable for the Practice and practical for the patient. Personally, I think patients should be able to book up at least two weeks ahead in order to be able to plan their lives.

Some Practices use nurse triage. You haven't mentioned this or telephone consultations.

I really don't know a lot about this. In my own Practice, I had sufficient capacity not to need triage, which in the past I have seen as a way of finding alternatives to seeing doctors. I now realise that this is not necessarily true. The experience with our nurse-led Minor Ailment Clinics indicated that patients might actually prefer to speak with nurse. This, however, would not be true nurse triage, but a telephone consultation with a nurse, which is a different matter altogether.

In fairness, I have not explored the possibilities around the use of the telephone in Practice. It was certainly something my Practice manager felt passionately about. I have decided to do some PDSA Cycles about the use of telephones, so I hope to be able to answer your question soon!

You said that every body that works in the Practice provides care. What did you mean in terms of receptionists?

My definition of care is whatever improves the lot of another and a carer as somebody who does this. Everybody who works in a General Practice, in some way or other, improves the lot of our patients.

More specifically, I can remember seeing an elderly spinster leaving Mercheford House one lunchtime and commenting on it to my secretary who regularly covered reception over the lunch hour.

"Oh she usually comes in once a week at this time. She knows I'm on the desk and likes to come in for a chat when she knows the place is quiet, and you're not around!"

Receptionists are often the first contact the patients have with the surgery. The style and content of this contact can improve or depress their mood.

Advanced access can affect your health – if your partners do not agree with what you doing. I have been trying to introduce Advanced Access into our Practice, but all I seem to get is another type of appointment, something which I know is self-defeating. It can be quite depressing. How do you cope with this?

I think there at least two comments I would make:

a) Being a change agent or causing change is a difficult role. It is not one that generally gets brownie points! It can be very lonely. People are defensive as they feel you are criticising them personally rather that the system in which they operate.

Change, nevertheless, starts from individuals, Keep going! Try to join up with someone else who shares your views, perhaps even in another Practice.

b) The second point is something about a shared vision, We've touched on this before. The fact of the matter is that unless the Practice as a whole has a clear and shared vision, it is unlikely that everybody necessary will be able to work together to sustain Advanced Access in the first place. The Government's access targets may help create a need for change, but will not in themselves effect the change.

People differ in their reaction to 'visions' – it depends partly on how they are motivated. In our Practice, I am conscious of 'selling visions' in different ways. Some folk can be enthused by a description of the 'Promised Land', and can quickly visualise new ideas and concepts. For others, this is a complete turn off; it terrifies them. Often they will respond to the notion of leading them away from their current difficulties. It boils down, I suppose, to the difference between leading 'to' and leading 'from'.

I agree that the circumstances you describe are difficult. Perhaps there is a colleague in your local Primary Care Development Team Centre with whom you can speak. If not, I am sure the National Primary Care Collaborative team would be able to put you in touch with a local kindred spirit.

You have not spent a lot of time on the arithmetic or measurement in delivering of Advance Access. Is there somewhere we can learn about this?

Fair comment. I have concentrated on the development of the concepts that support Advanced Access. Once you start asking questions of your own Practice and measuring activity in the areas

[1] Contact details: National Primary Care Development Team, Gateway House, Piccadilly South, Manchester M60 7LP. Tel: 0161 236 1566; Fax: 0161 236 4857; Email: npcdt@ manchester.nwest.nhs.uk; Web: www.npdt.org

around demand and supply, it should become fairly obvious what you should be doing.

For more exact details of the methodology promoted by The Primary Care Development Team you can do no better than to read John Oldham's booklet entitled *Advanced Access in Primary Care*.[1] He provides practical examples of the mathematics to which you refer.

How did you manage to get patients to go to your nurses instead of seeing you?

By explaining to them why it was a better way.

I have had an interest in hypertension for many years, especially hypertension in the elderly, and had a fairly large continuously screened population dependent on me for their long-term management. This constituted a significant personal workload. Having identified this, developed a protocol for the management of hypertension with our nurses, I simply invited patients to come to the Blood Pressure Clinic for their next BP check, rather than make an appointment with me.

This was difficult at first, but after trying different forms of words for my explanation, I become more comfortable with what I said (good time to use a PDSA Cycle!) When I explained that I was shifting routine work to the nurses so that I could make space to see them quickly when they really needed to see a doctor, they readily understood. This news soon got around; so much so that some patients began to get upset that they still had to come to see me!

Personally, I do not think informing patients of such changes should be delegated to reception staff, or others in the Practice, It is for the doctor to explain the changes in the way he operates; written leaflets personally given to patients help as well, but is best to come from the doctor.

We also use patient-held BP record cards which tell the patient when the nurse will refer the patient back to the doctor. The nurse also makes it clear that, when she is altering medication, she is doing so on the written instruction of the doctor. It is important to emphasise that the doctor and nurse work as a single team, sharing the care of individual patients.

In terms of asthma follow-up, the change over from doctor to nurse was probably easier in that:

1. Nurses' appointments ware longer than mine.
2. The visit to nurse was seen as adding value in that she had and did things that I did not normally do. For example, she had a

display of all the inhaler devices and performed spirometry, height and weight, PEFRs, etc.

3. I often bring her into a consultation and discuss the patient's long-term management with her in front of the patient. She is seen, has an opinion which I respect and one to which I take notice. It is then fairly simple for me to hand over follow-up to her, the Practice expert!

This last point is probably crucial: in the same way as patients are happy to be referred to consultant colleagues they know we respect, they are equally happy to see Practice colleagues when they know we respect them, I have not found transfer of care a problem.

In summary...

Writing a conclusion to a book like this is difficult, for many of its conclusions fly in the face of conventional wisdom and current opinion. It does seem counter-intuitive.

All I can say is that they have worked for Mercheford House. Life is not perfect; we still have hiccups, and we get it wrong from time to time; we still face many of the pressures of Primary Care in 2002; we are not conscious of having been resourced to achieve this.

What is true is that which I have reported has happened; it is true that patients are seen on the day they wish to be seen by their registered doctor and we do not have complaints about access.

Advanced Access is an essentially 'people thing' – it springs from values and cultures inherent in the Practice. It is not simply a series of processes – it is an example of whole systems thinking. It is something that is empowering and rewarding, and I recommend it to all!

References

Open Access

Do Patients Love You, but Hate Your Phones?; Helen Lippman, *Medical Economics,* September 18, 2000, pp. 77–84. (www.memag.com)
http://me.pdr.net/me/public.htm?path=content/journals/m/data/2000/0918/foneflow.html

Modernizing the NHS. Patient Care: Access; Mark Murray; *British Medical Journal,* June 10, 2000, Vol. 320, 1594–6. (www.bmj.com)

Same-Day Appointments: Exploding the Access Paradigm; Mark Murray MD, MPA and Catherine Tantau BSN, MPA, *Family Practice Management,* September 2000, pp. 45–50 (www.aafp.org)
http://www.aafp.org/fpm/20000900/45same.html

Same-Day Scheduling; Helen Lippman, *Hippocrates* February 2000, pp. 49–53. (www.hippocrates.com)
http://www.hippocrates.com/archive/February2000/02features/02openaccess.html

You mean I can see the doctor today?; DA Grandinetti; *Medical Economics,* March 20, 2000, pp. 102–114 (www.memag.com)
http://me.pdr.net/me/public.htm?path=content/journals/m/data/2000/0320/sameday.html

Presentations

Eastern Region Access Collaborative, Learning Session Two, 31 October and 1 November 2001

Mark Murray's presentation on *Redesign the System*
http://www.doh.gov.uk/ero/accesscollaborative/learningsessions/lsessiontwo/ls2.htm

Other Access References may be found on the ERO Access Collaborative Website
http://www.doh.gov.uk/ero/accesscollaborative/learningsessions/lsessiontwo/general/references.htm

Texts

Theory of Constraints; Eliyahu M Goldratt. 1990. North River Press.
Breakthrough Thinking; 1994. Gerald Nadlar and Sozo Hibino. Prima Publishing.
Advanced Access in Primary Care. 2001. John Oldham.
Management Teams; 2000. R. Meredith Belbin.
Harvard Business Review on Change: Leading Change: Why Transformation Efforts Fail, 1991. John P. Kotter.
The Tao of Coaching, 1997. Max Landsberg. Harper Collins Business
The Little Book of Coaching, 2002. Ken Blanchard and Don Shula. Harper Collins Business.

Websites

National Primary Care Collaborative
http://www.npdt.org

NHS Modernisation Agency
http://www.modernnhs.nhs.uk

Institute for Healthcare Improvement
http://www.ihi.org